Drugs into Bodies

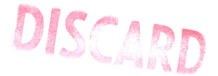

Drugs into Bodies
Global AIDS Treatment Activism

Raymond A. Smith and Patricia D. Siplon

Afterword by Alan Berkman

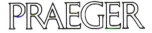 PRAEGER

Westport, Connecticut
London

362.196
S657d

Library of Congress Cataloging-in-Publication Data

Smith, Raymond A., 1967–
Drugs into Bodies: global AIDS treatment activism/Raymond A.
Smith and Patricia D. Siplon; afterword by Alan Berkman.
    p. ; cm.
Includes bibliographical references and index.
ISBN 0-275-98325-0 (alk. paper)
1. AIDS (Disease)–Social aspects. 2. AIDS (Disease)–Chemotherapy.
3. Community health services–Cross-cultural studies.
4. AIDS (Disease)–Patients–Services for–Cross-cultural studies.
I. Siplon, Patrica D. II. Title.
[DNLM: 1. Acquired Immunodeficiency Syndrome–drug discovery.
2. HIV Infections–drug therapy. 3. Health Services Accessibility.
4. International Cooperation. 5. Politics. WC 503.2 S657d 2006]
RA643.8.S65 2006
362.196'9792–dc22   2005034798

British Library Cataloguing in Publication Data is available.

Library of Congress Catalog Card Number: 2005034798
ISBN 0-275-98325-0 (alk. paper)

First published in 2006

Praeger Publishers, 88 Post Road West, Westport, CT 06881
An imprint of Greenwood Publishing Group, Inc.
www.praeger.com

Printed in the United States of America

The paper used in this book complies with the
Permanent Paper Standard issued by the National
Information Standards Organization (Z39.48–1984).

10 9 8 7 6 5 4 3 2 1

Contents

Preface

"Drugs into Bodies!" This simple slogan is just one of the many that have been shouted at AIDS demonstrations, emblazoned on T-shirts, and printed on placards. Yet perhaps more than any other slogan, it encapsulates the central challenge that has faced activists seeking to promote access to effective and affordable treatments for HIV.

For the first fifteen years of the AIDS epidemic, the emphasis was on the first half of the slogan: *drugs*. Between 1981 and 1996, there were simply no medications available that could effectively stop the spread of HIV in the human body or slow the progression of HIV infection to what is often called "full-blown AIDS." Although there was broad agreement on the importance of producing such medications, many people viewed this as solely a technical scientific problem unrelated to politics and certainly not susceptible to political pressure.

Others, however, recognized that scientific research is itself embedded in social, cultural, and political contexts. They saw sclerotic bureaucracies, inertial policymaking, inadequate funding, archaic scientific procedures, societal indifference, government hostility, corporate greed, absent leadership, and many other human-made impediments to scientific progress—all of which could be susceptible to political pressure even if the virus itself was not. And so was born AIDS treatment activism, a movement focused mostly in the developed world, and particularly in the United States, where the resources existed that might lead to effective drug development.

This domestic movement combined key strengths—unprecedented media savvy, uniquely postmodern sensibilities, and the accumulated lessons of previous civil rights movements—with the relentless focus of those who were literally fighting for their lives. Domestic AIDS treatment activists, especially the protest group ACT UP, radically altered the nation's system for accessing health care and redefined the doctor-patient relationship, the clinical trials system, the drug-approval process, and much more, often setting powerful precedents for other activists who have followed.

After the introduction of effective anti-HIV drug combinations in 1996, the emphasis of AIDS treatment activism shifted to the second part of the slogan: *into bodies*. In the developed world, this problem of treatment access was far less acute than the initial challenge of developing drugs. Most of the affluent countries of the world had systems of universal health care that provided access to new antiretroviral drugs as they became available. In the absence of universal coverage, the United States developed a network of AIDS Drug Assistance Programs (ADAPs), which, while imperfect and incomplete, expanded treatment access to thousands of impoverished citizens.

But in the poorer countries of the world, home to the vast majority of people with HIV, only a tiny percentage of the most elite had access to the drugs that could save the lives of millions. With drug regimens priced at between ten and fifteen thousand dollars per person annually, impoverished countries with per capita incomes of just a few hundred dollars and minimal public health infrastructures could never hope to treat their ever-growing populations of the sick and dying. It appeared to many that the problem of providing wide-ranging access to drugs would run aground on the ironclad laws of economics as surely as the problem of drug development had been thwarted by the laws of biology and chemistry.

But once again, a handful of activists and public health professionals saw that many of the principal impediments to global access to HIV medications were human-made, even more so than had been the case during the era of drug development before 1996. They discovered that the prices charged by pharmaceutical companies bore almost no relation to the actual cost of production or even to the recouping of research and development expenses, but were based purely on a desire for maximum profits. And they realized to their disgust that the pharmaceutical companies could easily have allowed generic versions of their medications to be produced at a tiny fraction of the prices they charged, almost instantly alleviating the world's most devastating health crisis.

Instead the pharmaceutical giants filed lawsuits under international trade agreements to protect their patents and convinced global institutions and powerful governments, especially the United States, to threaten developing countries with crippling economic sanctions. Yet most perversely of all, allowing generic drug development would scarcely have cost the pharmaceutical companies a cent; so few drugs were being sold in the developing world that there were virtually no profits being made there. Instead, the position of the pharmaceutical companies was based on a fear of "blowback"—the concern that revealing the true cost of production and lowering the costs of drugs in one part of the world would expose the exorbitantly inflated prices they charged in the developed world. Consigning millions of people to excruciating deaths and driving entire nations into shattering poverty was of less concern than protecting the profit margins that made pharmaceutical manufacturing one of the planet's most lucrative industries.

Of course, the developed world has long shown an enormous capacity to overlook, ignore, or explain away the suffering of the developing world. Malnutrition remains widespread, for instance, and easily treatable conditions such as tuberculosis, malaria, and enteric diseases cause countless deaths each year. But in the case of HIV infection, there was one crucial difference—there were a core of committed activists in the developed world who were engaged and mobilized around the issue of AIDS in ways that they were not around other diseases. These activists, primarily in the United States and Western Europe, could draw upon more than a decade of their own experience in combating AIDS in their own countries while also linking up with activists from developing countries who had begun working in parallel. And so was born the second great AIDS treatment activist movement, this one focused principally on promoting access to drugs in the developing world but involving a dense global network of activist organizations in both the global North and South.

Drugs into Bodies: Global AIDS Treatment Activism takes as its task the analysis of the rise, and remarkable success, of this second great AIDS treatment activist movement. The scope of the book is very much defined, then, by the key terms "activism" and "treatment." By activism, we refer to "contentious politics"—the process by which less empowered groups contend with powerful interests via such tactics as protests, demonstrations, direct actions, and other confrontational tactics. We recognize, and at times discuss, the many other types of activities that have also had a major impact on the promotion of access to AIDS treatments, including policymaking work, academic studies, interest group lobbying, the arts, and philanthropy. But our principal focus remains on "activism" in the form of contentious politics, in part because it uniquely intersects with all of these areas and because it has in many ways been the engine driving the response to global AIDS.

Similarly, the struggle against AIDS has been fought on many fronts, including HIV prevention, care provision, protection of personal privacy, vaccine development, women's and minority rights, poverty alleviation, and stigma reduction. Although all of these and many other aspects are crucially important in their own right, we believe that treatment has been central for at least three reasons. First, many of those most mobilized around AIDS treatment issues have been individuals who are themselves living with or directly affected by HIV, adding a greater sense of urgency to questions of treatment. Second, given the vast numbers of people infected with HIV, treatment presents the most compelling and immediate need; effective treatments can additionally have important effects on other areas such as the empowerment of people with HIV and the success of prevention programs. Third, treatment has been the arena in which it has been possible to achieve relatively broad agreement; many groups may disagree on various approaches to HIV prevention or women's rights, for instance, but few disagree in principle about the desirability of treating sick people.

Finally, our emphasis is on AIDS treatment activism in the era of globalization. The availability of effective antiretroviral drug combinations happened to coincide almost exactly with two of the foundational events of modern globalization: the launching of the World Trade Organization (WTO) and the enactment of the Trade-Related Aspects of Intellectual Property (TRIPS) Agreement. These two events drastically reshaped the context within which global trade is conducted, making it dramatically more difficult for poorer countries to obtain affordable access to patented anti-HIV drugs than might have been the case ten or even five years earlier. Of necessity, then, any examination of the challenge of securing access to HIV treatments can only be discussed against the backdrop of processes of globalization.

This volume is organized into two parts. Part I was authored primarily by Raymond A. Smith and focuses on AIDS treatment activism in the United States. Chapter 1 offers an analysis of the emergence of the first wave of AIDS treatment activism in the United States. Beginning with the first identification in 1981 of what was later to become known as AIDS, the chapter focuses in particular on the emergence and growth of the protest group ACT UP in 1987 through its sharp decline after 1992. Although they occurred before the start of the contemporary era of globalization, the events recounted in Chapter 1 set essential precedents and established key networks that shaped subsequent developments. This chapter also presents a recounting of AIDS treatment activism in the United States before 1996 and can stand alone in that regard. Chapter 2 picks up in 1996 and traces the development of a globally oriented treatment activist movement in the United States, a second activist wave that was distinct from but very much rooted in the first wave. Its emphasis is on the years 1998 and 1999, when a new coalition called Health GAP was launched. Although Health GAP was by no means the only early actor in the global treatment access movement, we focus on it because it, in a unique way, continued the work of ACT UP at the global level and because its base in the United States enabled it to quickly assume a leading activist role at the global level. The organization of both of these chapters draws heavily from the "political process model" of social movement development. This model was first introduced in 1982 by sociologist Doug McAdam and has been articulated for more than two decades through an ever-growing body of literature in political science and sociology, to which this volume represents a new contribution.[1]

Part II of the book, chiefly authored by Patricia D. Siplon, shifts the focus to the global arena. Bookended by an International AIDS Conference and a special session of the United Nations, Chapter 3 chronicles the eventful twelve-month period from mid-2000 to mid-2001. During this seemingly brief window of time, Health GAP and a collection of largely independent national and international organizations coalesced into a coordinated, if not quite unified, global AIDS treatment access movement. Chapter 4 picks up the narrative in the immediate aftermath of the September 11 attacks. Chronicling events through to 2005, this chapter traces new barriers to the movement created by the post–September 11 political environment, as well as the paradoxical challenge faced by the treatment access movement created by its winning its key demands. Part II continues to draw upon the McAdam political process model, but also is informed by more recent scholarship by its Margaret Keck and Kathleen Sikkink on the formation of "transnational issue advocacy networks," of which the global AIDS treatment activist movement is an important new example.[2]

The volume concludes with an Afterword by one of the most eloquent and influential figures in the struggle against global AIDS, longtime activist and Health GAP founder Alan Berkman. A visionary of the first order, Berkman offers his views of the challenges ahead in a battle against AIDS whose conclusion sadly remains as far out of sight as ever.

Acknowledgments

This book is the culmination of three years of collaboration by the authors, beginning in the aftermath of the American Political Science Association annual meeting in 2002. Both of the authors had begun their work on AIDS in their capacity as academic political scientists, but over time became drawn also to applied work in public policy, advocacy, and direct service. Reflecting our dual interests as academics and activists, it is our hope that this volume will have some impact on both in the academic and applied spheres.

Ray Smith's work has been at the community and grassroots level in New York City as well as at the policy level in Washington DC. Ray wishes to thank his colleagues at the variety of institutions at which he has worked over the past decade, including the Columbia University Department of Political Science, the HIV Center for Clinical and Behavioral Studies at the New York State Psychiatric Institute, the community-based agency Body Positive of New York, and the National Alliance of State and Territorial AIDS Directors (NASTAD) in Washington DC. For support and assistance on this book, he is in particular grateful to Alan Berkman, Alex Carballo-Dieguez, Theo Sandfort, David Hoos, Kim Johnson, Shareen Hertel, and Rainer Braun of Columbia University; Sharonann Lynch and Paul Davis of Health GAP; John James of *AIDS Treament News;* Mark Milano of ACT UP New York; Hilary Claggett and Gary Kuris of Praeger Publishers; and, of course, coauthor Trish Siplon.

Trish Siplon has been an AIDS scholar and activist since the early 1990s, and joined Health GAP as a Core Volunteer in December 2000. She would like to thank her mentors at the AIDS Action Committee in Boston, where she volunteered during graduate school. She is also grateful to her current colleagues at Saint Michael's College in Vermont, as well as at the Department of Political Science at the University of Dar es Salaam in Tanzania, which graciously hosted her during 2002 and fall semester 2005. She is particularly grateful to the two sets of AIDS treatment activists with whom she has worked most closely, her students at Saint Michael's College and the staff and fellow volunteers of Health GAP. For their work during the writing of this book, she would especially like to thank former and current students Jessica Bassett, Ashley George, Dusty Haselton, Jamila Headley, Michael McCarthy, Erin McDonnell, and Rob Mealey, and SGAC coadvisors Michael Bosia and Cliff Lubitz. As for the activists within Health GAP, they collectively represent a truly awe-inspiring collectivity of talent and commitment, and Trish would like to individually thank all the members but especially Brook Baker, founder Alan Berkman, T. Richard Corcoran, David Hoos, Donnarae Palmer, Eustacia Smith, and Rob Weissman, as well as the three members of the indefatigable staff who have stayed with the organization since it was founded: Paul Davis, Sharonann Lynch, and Asia Russell. She would also like to recognize the contributions of another of Health GAP's early volunteers, Evan Ruderman, who died in November 2003. She was a wonderful friend, and the way she lived her life is a powerful model for the activist and PWA communities to which she contributed so much. Finally, her greatest thanks are reserved for the two people who showed the most patience with her during the writing process, her husband Todd Watkins and coauthor Ray Smith.

Part I

Building a Domestic AIDS Treatment Activist Movement

Introduction

When AIDS was first identified in 1981, it seemed to appear as much out of a clear sky as a meteor strike, something that was simply not there one moment and then inescapably there the next. More than two decades of research have yet to produce conclusive results about how, when, and where HIV first came to infect human beings. But it is now clear that the spread of the virus has been deeply embedded in larger social, economic, and political processes. The journey from HIV as an infection among small primates in the Central African jungle to a mortal threat to more than 40 million people in every corner of the world can only be understood in a larger context stretching over at least fifty years. Post-World War II decolonization and migrant workforces laboring under apartheid; refugee flows after civil wars and modern mass transportation linking the world's urban centers; changes in the social and sexual organization of society and the proliferation of the global narcotics trade—the spread of HIV cannot be mapped without reference to these and countless other broad global socioeconomic processes.

Just as it is easy to view the emergence of AIDS as a bolt from the blue, so too it is tempting to think of the *response* to AIDS as equally constructed out of thin air. In order to meet the demands of the epidemic, entirely new scientific subfields and biomedical specialities have been developed, novel terms and concepts have been coined, and a seemingly unprecedented breed of activism has been born in the heat of the battle against the virus. Yet just as the spread of the virus can only be understood in terms of larger and longer-term processes, so too the response to AIDS must be viewed through a wider lens.

Part I of this book seeks to provide that wider lens. Chapter 1 traces the systematic progression of reactions to the new disease from overwhelmed shock to outraged anger to effective mobilization. The focus in this chapter is on the United States, the country in which the epidemic was first identified and in which the first and largest sustained response was mounted. At the heart of Chapter 1 are the circumstances leading up to the explosive founding and furious activity of the protest group ACT UP, especially at its height in the years between 1987 and 1992. Although AIDS activism is larger and more encompassing that just ACT UP, that group is widely acknowledged to have been the flagship of AIDS activist efforts, particularly with regard to treatment issues.

In Chapter 2, the timeframe shifts to the late 1990s and the lens is widened further. By 1998, it had become apparent that the vast majority of people in the developing world were being denied access to the lifesaving antiretroviral drugs introduced in the developed world in 1996. In response to the need to "bridge the gap" in access to treatment, a new response was mounted by activists, among them a group that came to be called Health GAP. Chapter 2 recounts how a small but dedicated group drew on pre-existing networks and proven strategies from ACT UP and other organizations to launch a protest movement that would begin to move U.S. public policy with astonishing speed.

THE POLITICAL PROCESS MODEL

It was by no means a foregone conclusion that an effective activist effort would emerge to combat AIDS either domestically or globally, and certainly not assured that these movements would emerge at the particular time and in the particular form that they did. Indeed, of all the types of collective action that could be organized in response to all the grievances that exist in the world, only a relative few ever manage to coalesce into forces to be reckoned with. Yet some movements do from time to time originate within society in opposition to the action of states and other powerful forces. Such "social movements" have become increasingly important parts of the political landscape in both the United States and abroad. This has presented political science, sociology, and other related fields with the challenge of understanding and explaining why some movements successfully emerge, how they substantially achieve their goals, and why most vary over time in effectiveness, often eventually declining or disintegrating entirely.

The organization of Part I draws upon the "political process model" of social movement emergence that was introduced in 1982 by political sociologist Doug McAdam.[1]

This new model was introduced in response to limitations that McAdam perceived in two other existing models of social movement development, one that emphasized the role of psychological factors and another emphasizing the mobilization of resources. The political process model incorporates elements of these two earlier models, but broadens the framework to include more factors that interact with one another in more complex ways. The model was developed with particular reference to the Civil Rights Movement in the American South, but has been adapted to apply to many other contexts, and is also broadly applicable to the case of AIDS treatment activism.

McAdam's model begins with the observation that social movements do not emerge in a matter of days or weeks in response to abrupt changes, but are deeply rooted in *broad socioeconomic processes* that are often quite unrelated to the grievances of any particular social movement. In the case of the Civil Rights Movement, for instance, he argued that that the mechanization of agriculture in the rural South and the concurrent development of synthetic fibers drastically diminished the demand for agricultural workers in cotton fields. At about the same time, changes in federal immigration law largely shut off the supply of new immigrant labor at a time when the expanding factories of many northern cities needed increasing numbers of workers. The confluence of these and other factors helped to trigger the great migration of African Americans into northern states where they also happened to have the right to vote, resulting for the first time in a significant number of black voters in the United States.

Broad socioeconomic processes can also often lead to changes in *political opportunities*. Although disadvantaged groups remain weak, windows of time may open up during which they gain strength relative to the dominant forces that seek to continue to oppress or marginalize them. Thus, for instance, black voters in the North became an integral component of the New Deal Coalition that helped to ensure the election first of Franklin Delano Roosevelt and then of Harry Truman. With liberals in the White House continuously between 1933 and 1953, economic policies were passed to alleviate poverty (which was at its worst among blacks), the armed forces were integrated, and liberal judges were appointed to the federal judiciary (including to the Supreme Court that would strike down segregation in 1954).

The simple opening of a window of political opportunity is not enough, however, in the McAdam model. Many such windows briefly open and then are snapped shut again when a disadvantaged population does not manage to seize the moment. In order to succeed, groups must make the most of *mobilizing structures* (also called "indigenous organizational strength") that originate within the group, such as preexisting social networks that allow for coordinated action and home-grown leaders who can act with high levels of credibility. Ironically, in the case of the civil rights movement, segregation in some ways actually intensified the ability of southern blacks to form dense networks based in the all-black institutions and locales in which they were required to spend their lives.

As crucial as political opportunities and mobilizing structures are, however, they are insufficient alone. They also require a "spark" to ignite them, a process that McAdam calls *cognitive liberation*. "While important, expanding political opportunities and indigenous organizations do not, in any simple sense, produce a social movement," notes McAdam (p. 49). "In the absence of one other crucial process these two factors remain necessary, but insufficient, causes of insurgency. Together they offer insurgents a certain objective 'structural potential' for collective political action. Mediating between opportunity and action are people and the subjective meanings they attach to their situations," that is to say, whether they have experienced cognitive liberation.

As the name suggests, cognitive liberation (also called "cultural framing") refers to the ways in which people are able to emancipate their way of thinking about their circumstances. Cognitive liberation has at least three distinct stages, during which individuals and communities come to believe that (1) the status quo is illegitimate; (2) the status quo could be changed; and (3) they as individuals and as a community can effect this change. Infused alongside these ways of *thinking* are also ways of *feeling*; emotion and affect are an inseparable part of the framing of a situation. Thus in the civil rights movement, the relative empowerment of African Americans in the North and the ongoing support of the White House and the federal judiciary, among other social and political factors, began to make the possibility of change seem real and to embolden feelings of hope. Crucial early successes in the South, most notably the Montgomery bus boycott, then reinforced the sense that southern blacks could be the instruments of their own emancipation, further building indigenous organizational strength and allowing political opportunities to be maximized.

AIDS TREATMENT ACTIVISM AND THE POLITICAL PROCESS MODEL

The political process model thus provides a powerful interpretive framework through which to examine other significant social movements. This would include the development of a domestically oriented, and then later of a globally oriented, AIDS treatment activist movement in the United States. The goal of Part I of this book is to explain how these two movements came into being, and to identify the continuities and discontinuities between them. Part I also seeks to contribute an important new case study to the burgeoning literature on social movement emergence and development.

Chapter 1 discusses a range of seemingly unconnected *broad socioeconomic processes*—including the antibiotics revolution, the rise of a gay and lesbian movement, and the Reagan-era shift toward social and political conservatism—that all framed the issue of AIDS in the United States during the 1980s. Chapter 2 examines a different set of broad socioeconomic factors, most notably the uncontrolled spread of HIV in sub-Saharan Africa at a time when processes of globalization were leading to the maximization of patent protections and hence of supremacy of profits over even critical public health and humanitarian concerns.

Changing *political opportunities* are also key to understanding the growth of AIDS activism. McAdam argues that a new social movement may have opportunities for action whenever the position of challengers becomes stronger relative to that of the dominant group. For AIDS activism, windows of political opportunity opened in particular during two crucial years. Chapter 1 hinges on the key year of 1987, in which the general population of the United States was finally becoming concerned about AIDS and in which AIDS activists at last found a strong and effective voice via the protest group ACT UP. In Chapter 2, the pivotal year is 1999, when the presidential run of a sitting U.S. vice president and the stirrings of a militant antiglobalization movement provided crucial openings for action on the international front.

Of course, when political opportunities arise, they are sometimes lost because groups lack the *mobilizing structures* to form networks or to produce effective leadership. Chapter 1 explains the ways in which domestic AIDS activism was largely made possible by dense networks among gay men in major cities and by an ideology that decentralized organizational authority and made "every member a leader." Chapter 2 examines the rapid emergence and early successes of globally focused activism beginning in 1999 as a product of the networks created through the domestic AIDS activism of a decade earlier in concert with public health practitioners and nongovernmental organizations keenly aware of the threats posed by global AIDS.

Regarding AIDS activism, *cognitive liberation* was often born out of desperation among people who felt that their lives hung in the balance. Chapter 1 recounts how over a span of six years tentative steps toward self-empowerment ultimately culminated in cognitive liberation once activists made a commitment to "act up." Chapter 2 outlines a quicker process of constructing a global agenda, one that was emboldened by the successes of the domestic movement, which had proven that change is possible.

   The political process model also helps to explain how a social movement functions after its initial emergence. Broad socioeconomic processes continue to play an important background role, but can either promote or hinder the work of the movement. Political opportunities also continue to shift, often turning against a social movement once its opponents manage to rally their own strengths and find ways to undermine or co-opt the movement. Mobilizing structures may also splinter, as fatigue and infighting begin to set in. And the way that movement leaders and participants begin to understand their situation may also change, leading to a decline in consensus, a loss of focus, disagreement over goals and strategies, intramovement rivalries, and organizational fragmentation. Indeed, movements that appear to just be hitting their stride have often, in retrospect, already begun their decline. These themes are discussed in Chapter 1 as contributing to the virtual disintegration of ACT UP and the drop-off in domestic AIDS activism more generally after 1992. They are also addressed in Part II of the book with regard to potential threats to activist efforts to counter global AIDS.

Chapter 1

ACTION=LIFE: Responding to AIDS on the Home Front

When Albert Alexander began tending his rose garden one morning in 1941, he had no idea that he would be making medical history. An Oxford police constable, Alexander nicked himself with a thorn but thought little more of it until the cut became infected. Soon, his face became swollen and his body temperature rocketed to 105 degrees. Bacteria had entered his bloodstream, causing septicemia, and in 1941 people whose own immune systems could not combat septicemia faced death—treatments were nonexistent. Alexander was brought to the Radcliffe Hospital in London, where his doctors judged that he had only a few hours to live and requested permission to administer an experimental substance called penicillin. Although Alexander later died, his treatment marked the start of the "antibiotics revolution." Subsequent patients survived thanks to penicillin, and mass production of antibiotics was then undertaken, saving untold numbers of lives during World War II and beyond. Whereas humans were once completely at the mercy of bacteria, antibiotics had the ability to kill the bacteria that caused many fearsome infections.[1]

In the decades following the antibiotics revolution, people in the affluent countries of the world would become accustomed to the idea that people do not die from small nicks and cuts, or even usually from large-scale infections such as pneumonia, tuberculosis, and meningitis. In the 1960s and 1970s, antibiotics met up with the birth-control pill, changing social mores, and a demographic surge of Baby Boomers to spawn a sexual revolution. During this period, rates of sexually transmitted diseases (STDs) skyrocketed, but bacterial STDs such as syphilis and gonorrhea could be easily cured by antibiotics. STDs of viral origin, however, were invulnerable to such treatments, with two emerging as especially problematic: genital herpes and hepatitis B. But despite being termed a modern Scarlet

Letter, genital herpes turned out to be incurable and stigmatizing but not usually a major health hazard, with medications developed to suppress outbreaks. Likewise, in the mid-1970s, researchers undertook vaccine studies among gay male communities, whose members were disproportionately infected with the hepatitis B virus. After vigorous outreach and intensive study, a vaccine was successfully developed that conferred effective and long-lasting immune protection against hepatitis B in almost all who received it.

Yet perhaps the greatest triumph of biomedicine and public health came with the 1977 eradication of smallpox. One of the deadliest viruses in history, smallpox has been circulating in human populations throughout the world since prehistoric times. Although a vaccine was developed in the eighteenth century using the closely related cowpox virus, it was not until 1966 that teams from the World Health Organization (WHO) set out to systematically vaccinate the global population. These roving teams ultimately reached hundreds of millions of individuals and, in the process, left ever-fewer hosts for the virus. By December 1979, the WHO was able to issue a proclamation certifying that smallpox had been eradicated from the world.[2]

Thus by the start of the 1980s, broad socioeconomic processes, including scientific advances, had led to a point at which it seemed that the long struggle of humans against infectious disease had been all but won through a combination of advances in antibiotics, vaccine development, and epidemiological techniques. Indeed, much of the global biomedical establishment began to reorient its attention from battling contagions to fighting chronic ailments such as cancer, diabetes, and cardiovascular disease, which were proving increasingly common in affluent societies. Fewer steps were being taken to be vigilant for newly emerging diseases, and any challenges that might emerge were considered likely to be vanquished quickly by new medications, vaccinations, improved public health systems, and other scientific advances.

The world was thus ill-prepared for the short, nondescript article entitled "*Pneumocystis* Pneumonia—Los Angeles" that appeared in the June 5, 1981, edition of *Morbidity and Mortality Weekly Report (MMWR)*, a publication of the Centers for Disease Control and Prevention (CDC).[3] "In the period October 1980–May 1981, five young men, all active homosexuals, were treated for biopsy-confirmed *Pneumocystis carinii* pneumonia (PCP) at three different Los Angeles hospitals... *Pneumocystis* pneumonia in the United States is almost exclusively limited to severely immunosuppressed patients." The fact that all five men were homosexuals suggested a link to particular behaviors, the articled noted, and several had also suffered from heretofore unusual diseases such as esophageal and oral candidiasis, Hodgkin's disease, and cytomegalovirus infection.

A month later, *MMWR* reported that in the previous thirty months, twenty-six young gay men had been diagnosed with an aggressive form of a skin malignancy, Kaposi's sarcoma (KS), formerly found in much milder form among older men of Jewish and Mediterranean descent.[4] By late summer 1981, the contours of a full-blown epidemic were already coming into view. The August 28 issue of *MMWR* reported that an additional seventy cases of KS and PCP had been diagnosed. The illness would, of course, soon come to be called Acquired Immunodeficiency Syndrome, or AIDS, and somewhat more slowly be recognized as the late stage of infection with the bloodborne pathogen that would eventually be named the human immunodeficiency virus (HIV).

In retrospect, it is clear that many thousands of people must have already been infected with HIV by 1981, and some number had undoubtedly already died of AIDS. The early infections and deaths were clustered in particular among gay men, especially those with a "fast-lane" lifestyle and many sexual partners, because unprotected anal sex is an especially efficient route of viral transmission. Despite this concentration within a particular subculture, the new syndrome defied early identification for a variety of reasons. Without treatment, the time from initial HIV infection to the onset of serious symptoms averaged about ten years, delinking the illness from specific sexual or drug-related risk behaviors that had occurred long before. The early symptoms of immune suppression are also highly nonspecific and sometimes not especially severe—night sweats, swollen lymph nodes, gastrointestinal disorders, and neurological problems that could be ignored or explained by other causes.

Likewise, it would not usually be HIV infection itself that would directly contribute to illness. Rather, HIV infection most often would present opportunities for a host of other illnesses that would usually be kept in check by a healthy immune system. Indeed, more than two dozen cancers, fungal and bacterial infections, and other distinct conditions would eventually come to be regarded as "AIDS-defining illnesses," meaning that their presence in a person with HIV would lead to an official AIDS diagnosis. Thus, although AIDS had a unique power to ravage its victims, the disparate cluster of AIDS-related symptoms and conditions could not be identified as a distinct clinical entity, or syndrome, until enough similar cases emerged in the same time and place, as first happened in Los Angeles in 1981. Once AIDS was clearly identified, however, it was quickly diagnosed in an ever-mounting number of people. By February 1983, just over 1,000 AIDS diagnoses had been made and nearly 400 deaths counted; by the end of that year, both of those statistics had tripled. By the end of 1984, the number of Americans known to be living with or to have died from AIDS totaled nearly 8,000.[5]

Because AIDS eventually became a higher priority in the United States, it may be hard to remember that its gravity was largely discounted at the outset, even among some of the hardest-hit communities. Wary of pronouncements from a government that continued to persecute them, gay communities tended to view the idea of a fatal sexually transmitted disease with skepticism, suspecting yet another ploy to deny them sexual liberation. A pattern of deep denial about the sexual transmission of HIV set in among gay male communities, stoked in part because the influential owners of gay bars, clubs, and bathhouses were afraid of losing customers. Pessimism about AIDS also ran counter to a generally prevailing mood of progress and spirit of defiance to the then-new "religious right" coming to power under newly elected President Ronald Reagan. The editor of the gay newsmagazine *The Advocate* had even gone so far as to write in the first editorial of 1980 that "I foresee that the next ten years will be the best in the history of humankind."[6]

Mainstream society was also only too glad to remain silent on a disease that afflicted undesirables such as gay men, "drug addicts," and sex workers and involved discussing unsavory topics such as anal sex, gay bathhouses, heroin addiction, and bloody syringes. *The New York Times,* for instance, had printed only six articles by the end of 1982, none of them on the front page. This is in contrast to sixty-two articles, including eleven on the front page, on the comparatively minor 1976 outbreak of the respiratory infection called Legionnaire's disease, which killed 29 people and made 182 sick. AIDS did not break on the front page of *The New York Times* until May 25, 1983, at which point there had been some 1,450 known cases of AIDS.[7]

Although the reasons for this early apathy were many, no small part was due to a widespread belief that in the age of antibiotics, AIDS would be vanquished fairly quickly and easily. And there were, indeed, a number of major scientific breakthroughs in the first few years of the epidemic. Within a year of the epidemic's emergence, the main pathways of HIV transmission (sexual, bloodborne, and mother-to-child) had been determined, although the task of implementing effective preventive measures proved to be a much more difficult one. By 1983, it had been established that the causative agent behind AIDS was a previously unknown retrovirus, a type of virus that stores its genetic information on strands of RNA rather than the usual DNA. This new retrovirus, it was soon determined, primarily infected and destroyed a type of white blood cells, CD4 cells, which are essential components of the immune system. In 1985, a blood test was licensed to detect HIV antibodies, allowing individuals to learn whether they were infected. But while these advances in basic science were crucial building blocks, they alone provided little therapeutic value, a fact that was widely disregarded in favor of wishful thinking about quick progress. The most infamous such incident took place on April 23, 1984, when Secretary of Health and Human Services Margaret Heckler held a press conference to announce the discovery of the virus that would later be named HIV. "Today we add another miracle to the long honor roll of American medicine and science. Today's discovery represents the triumph of science over a dreaded disease," said Heckler, before incorrectly predicting that a blood test would be ready within six month and that vaccine testing would begin within two years.[8] And why not, many asked, given that an ancient scourge like smallpox had just been certified as eradicated and that new vaccines had been developed for a range of infectious diseases?

CARING FOR THE SICK, MOURNING FOR THE DEAD

Despite optimism about an early cure, the facts on the ground in the second half of 1981 were that gay men were falling sick and dying in ever-larger numbers. The new syndrome was especially horrifying because it mainly struck seemingly healthy people in the prime years of their lives and caused severely debilitating conditions and often excruciating deaths. These losses were enormously compounded because they struck within close-knit urban communities such as San Francisco's Castro district and New York's Greenwich Village in which gay men were linked through ties of friendship, geographic proximity, work connections, neighborhood bonds, and sometimes sexual contacts.

Because the new syndrome was striking within such well-established social networks, the first organized response began with anecdotal discussions, especially among gay men. These began vaguely but with increasing intensity after the July 3, 1981, publication of a then routine but now famous article in *The New York Times* entitled "Rare Cancer Found in 40 Homosexuals" about the first cases of Kaposi's sarcoma. The 1989 film *Longtime Companion,* about the brutal toll of AIDS in the 1980s, perhaps best captured that first response to AIDS with a dramatization of that day in which gay men are depicted reading the *Times* and calling one another to discuss the new "rare cancer."[9] Some are alarmed, others are confused, still others dismiss the article as government propaganda. But even during those first days, some gay men report having thought back to friends or lovers who had died mysteriously in the 1970s, and many began to intuit that the epidemic might have deeper roots than was evident on the surface.

The picture was further complicated, and the breadth of the epidemic began to seem greater, with news of emerging AIDS cases among nongay groups. Recipients of blood transfusions and blood products, for instance, were among the early groups diagnosed. Some of these were individuals who received transfusions as part of surgical procedures or after injuries, but many were people with blood disorders such as hemophilia. This was yet another sad irony of scientific advance: for centuries, hemophiliacs had been prone to uncontrolled internal bleeding usually due to a lack of either of two blood coagulants, called Factor VIII or Factor IX. In the late 1960s it became possible for the first time to use blood fractionating technologies to produce Factor VIII and Factor IX concentrates that could be transfused into hemophiliacs in order to help their blood to clot and enabling them to live far more normal and productive lives. But these concentrates were derived from the pooled blood plasma from as many as 60,000 people, virtually guaranteeing that most of those who received such transfusions would become HIV infected. Further, because hemophilia is a genetically based disease, these HIV infections were disproportionately concentrated within extended families in which several members might become ill with AIDS-related symptoms.[10]

As a bloodborne virus, HIV also found its way into networks of injection drug users. Given harshly prohibitionist drug laws and the strict regulation of supplies of sterile syringes, the sharing of needles was often a practical necessity for people with addictions to heroin or other powerful injectable drugs. Among heavy regular users, an entire subculture was built up around the act of injecting in groups, through which supplies of drugs could be shared whenever available and users helped each other avoid painful drug withdrawal symptoms. Shooting up in the presence of others was also desirable because users could then rely on friends to help them in the case of an overdose or to help them through a bad reaction. HIV transmission among injecting drug users was also exacerbated by sexual activity, both among themselves and with paying clients. Indeed, all sex workers who had unprotected intercourse with large numbers of sexual partners, whether drug users or not, were another population highly vulnerable to the sexual transmission of HIV.

Thus there were several distinct networks within which AIDS first struck, but most were not quick to mobilize politically. Already marginalized by both law and circumstance, injecting drug users and sex workers had few options or opportunities for collective action. Among people with hemophilia, familial and other networks had served as a basis for effective organization in attempts to secure treatment services, but these networks had largely avoided contentious political action. Gay communities, on the other hand, had been highly engaged in contentious political action in the 1970s, and included some members who were well educated, professionally successful, socially well connected, and in possession of relatively high levels of disposable income. Yet even with such resource-rich networks, political activism did not at first come as the natural response to what were felt as intensely personal losses.

Instead, the initial wave of organizing revolved around providing emergency assistance in the form of hot meals, psychological support, pain management, help with household chores, and simple companionship. In some cases, these volunteers were the only people willing to help people with AIDS. Initial fears about the possibility of HIV transmission through casual contact led many otherwise responsible health and service providers to abandon their professionalism and refuse to treat patients with the disease, creating an even more compelling need for compassionate volunteers. And in some ways, volunteers who themselves had AIDS, or whose partners and friends did, knew from their firsthand experience as much as, or more than, those with formal medical training.

The first wave of AIDS organizing was typified by the Gay Men's Health Crisis (GMHC), founded in the fall of 1981 to provide care and support for the sick and dying. The group developed quickly by drawing upon already existing friendship, neighborhood, professional, and other networks that predated the epidemic. Ironically, the same dense web of connections among urban gay men that had been facilitating the spread of the virus and compounding the sense of mourning and loss also proved to be an effective network for mobilizing a response to the new epidemic. GMHC and then other organizations were able to call upon this network not only for time and money, but also for expertise: doctors, nurses, lawyers, business owners, fundraisers, public relations specialists, journalists, artists, and many other skilled professionals were among those contributing to the early response to AIDS.[11]

The slew of volunteers that emerged to support GMHC was drawn not so much from among those who were gravely ill but from among their friends and partners as well as the "worried well" who saw themselves as vulnerable to the new disease. As sociologist Philip Kayal described his own experiences as a GMHC volunteer, "I was surrounded by death and dying. AIDS volunteerism was central to the physical and social survival of the community and I needed to do something responsible and find an outlet for my rage. People were being abandoned, friends were dying, and their pain

(our tremendous losses) was being discounted. Little did I know that volun-
teering and being with people with AIDS would give me a chance to do
something rewarding, useful, and politically significant, all at the same
time."[12]

Although GMHC would eventually become a sprawling, multipurpose
organization, it was best known early on for its "buddy" programs, which
matched a healthy volunteer with a sick client. It was joined at first by only
a few similar groups such as the San Francisco AIDS Foundation and the
Boston-based AIDS Action Committee of Massachusetts. In the absence of
any effective treatments, or even a basic understanding of the causes of
AIDS, the emphasis of these and other groups was inevitably on palliative
care in a hospicelike setting: comforting the sick, caring for the dying, and
eventually mourning the dead. As the death tolls rose, private funerals were
soon supplemented by public candlelight vigils and other commemorative
services. Little time or energy was left to think about political organizing or
the "larger picture" of the gathering disaster, although an inchoate anger
was already forming. "As early as 1982, it looked like an entire generation
of gay men, my generation in particular, was going to be wiped out," wrote
Kayal. "But no one seemed capable or concerned about preventing it—
except two or three informed gay activists and doctors in New York and
San Francisco."[13]

TOWARD SELF-EMPOWERMENT

For two years, people with AIDS themselves were largely absent from
organizing roles because by the time they were diagnosed they were usually
already close to death. Over the course of 1981 and 1982, however,
awareness grew about the types of symptoms that characterized earlier stages
of HIV infection, such as persistently swollen lymph nodes, night sweats,
and fatigue; a new term—"ARC" or AIDS-Related Complex—was even
coined to describe the cluster of earlier symptoms (ARC has since been
replaced with terms such as early HIV infection). This recognition of earlier
symptoms made it possible for people with AIDS or ARC (called PWAs or
PWARCs) to identify themselves as such before they reached end-stage
illness.

Even in the earliest days, however, a few individuals, notably Bobbi
Campbell and Dan Turner of San Francisco, publicly announced their
status as people with AIDS. Campbell began writing a column for the
San Francisco Sentinel and served on the board of the new KS/AIDS Foun-
dation, always publicly wearing a button with the message "SURVIVE."
Turner gave public speeches with a three-point message telling other gay

men to "Stay Informed. Be cautious, but not paranoid. And be supportive." Campbell and Turner together convened a meeting that spawned "People with AIDS San Francisco," the first PWA group. In 1982, Michael Callan and Richard Berkowitz in New York formed a parallel group called "Gay Men with AIDS" and also joined meetings of a group of public health professionals and medical providers called the New York AIDS Network.[14]

By 1983, many gay men knew that although they had AIDS they were still well enough to be active participants in their own health care, and had begun to feel patronized. "New York PWAs and PWARCs began to express growing frustration at attending too many GMHC forums in which those of us with AIDS would sit silently in the audience and hear doctors, nurses, lawyers, insurance experts, and social workers tell us what it was like to have AIDS," wrote Callan and Turner.[15] "It seemed to occur to several of us simultaneously . . . that there was something wrong with this picture. The 'real experts,' we realized, weren't up there . . . The idea struck us like a bolt of lightning. Until then, it simply hadn't occurred to those of us in New York who were diagnosed that we could be anything more than passive recipients of the genuine care and concern of those who hadn't (yet) been diagnosed." The opening chapter of an organized PWA self-empowerment movement was launched shortly thereafter in May 1983 out of an impromptu meeting of PWAs in a hospitality suite in a Denver hotel at the Fifth Lesbian and Gay Health Conference, which included the Second National AIDS Forum. Discussion centered around a vision of PWA groups in all the major AIDS epicenters, as well as a national association to link them together. The group articulated four guiding principles for a new era of PWA self-empowerment, and as Callan and Turner wrote, they then "decided to storm the closing session and to present our demands. In a democratic fashion, we each declaimed one of the points until our whole list of recommendations and responsibilities had been publicly uttered for the first time."[16]

The four points came to be called The Denver Principles and came to serve as a founding text for PWA self-empowerment. The Preamble introduces a strident new tone, stating, "We condemn attempts to label us as 'victim,' which implies defeat, and we are only occasionally 'patients,' which implies passivity, and dependence upon the care of others. We are 'people with AIDS.'" The first point addresses health-care professionals, challenging them to come to grips with their own attitudes about AIDS and to treat people with AIDS as "whole people and address psychosocial issues as well as biophysical ones." The second point targets "all people," urging them to "support us in our struggle" and not to scapegoat or blame PWAs. The final point identifies various rights of people with AIDS, including rights to full and satisfying sexual and emotional lives, to access to quality medical treatment and social services without discrimination and with full explanations of treatments, privacy, and confidentiality, and finally "to die and to LIVE in dignity."[17]

It is the third point, however, that forms the nucleus of subsequent PWA organization. This point begins by urging PWAs to "form caucuses to choose their own representatives, to deal with the media, to choose their own agenda, and to plan their own strategies." It continues to urge PWAs to "be involved at every level of AIDS decisionmaking...[and to] be included in all AIDS forums with equal credibility." It also urges PWAs to practice safer sex and to inform potential sexual partners about their health status. In the aftermath of the Denver meeting, the participants returned to their home cities with the goal of creating local People with AIDS Coalitions (PWAC) as well as a National Association of People with AIDS (NAPWA).[18]

POLITICAL STIRRINGS

Although PWAC took a notably more strident tone than GMHC and other service providers, its agenda was still primarily inward looking and not overtly involved with engaging governmental institutions. It adapted elements of twelve-step programs, self-help groups, and psychological insights from works such as the stages-of-dying framework developed by Elizabeth Kubler-Ross.[19] But the prevailing sense was still one of a temporary state of siege, one that would hopefully pass quickly with the development of effective treatments or even a cure. Meanwhile, it remained a challenge just to get through each new day. "People were dying left and right, horrible deaths, and nobody knew why. The shock was incredible. People were trying to figure out so hard how to take care of the people they cared about, how to take care of themselves, how not to get sick, how to prevent people from dying, how to get services to people in every way, shape, and form," said lesbian activist and academic Maxine Wolfe. "The idea of doing anything else was overwhelming."[20]

One of the few voices clearly articulating a political agenda as early as 1983 was that of novelist and playwright Larry Kramer. A contrarian to the core, Kramer had spent the late 1970s railing against what he considered a culture of gay promiscuity and shallowness, most powerfully in a scorching novel called *Faggots* that had led some in the community to shun him. In 1981, he was one of the founders of GMHC, although he eventually left the group in one of the many conflicts that seemed to define his life. Yet Kramer emerged as the single most influential figure in the AIDS politics of the 1980s, consistently prescient, utterly uncompromising, and unfailingly controversial.

In a long article in the gay-oriented *New York Native* newspaper—entitled "1,112 and Counting" to mark the rising death toll—Kramer overtly criticized the failure of the gay community to organize in response to the epidemic. "Every straight person who is knowledgeable about the AIDS epidemic can't understand why gay men aren't marching on the White House. Over and over again, I hear from them, 'Why aren't you guys doing anything?,'" wrote Kramer. "Every politician I have spoken to has said to me confidentially, 'You guys aren't making enough noise. Bureaucracy only responds to pressure.'" Hoping to stoke that pressure, "I hope that we don't have to conduct sit-ins or tie up traffic or get arrested. I hope our city and our country will start to do something to help start saving us. But it is time for us to be perceived for what we truly are: an angry community and a strong community." Kramer concludes his jeremiad with a call to action: "It is necessary that we have a pool of at least three thousand people who are prepared to participate in demonstrations of civil disobedience . . . I am asking every gay person and every gay organization to canvass friends and members and make a count of the total number you can provide towards this pool of three thousand."[21]

Yet much to Kramer's frustration, his article drew attention but failed to spark a protest movement, a fact that is particularly surprising because the gay community had a long history of protest politics. Indeed, the modern movement for gay, lesbian, and bisexual equality was launched by an act of protest—the Stonewall Riots of June 1969, during which customers of a gay bar in New York City fought back against a police raid. This act of resistance ignited not just three nights of street fighting but three decades of activism marked by targeted demonstrations and annual large-scale "pride marches" in most major U.S. cities. During the 1970s, groups such as the Gay Liberation Front and the Gay Activist Alliance had led protests and demonstrations, but by mid-decade they had moved away from their more confrontational tactics. This was in part due to the ebbing of the ethos of the "sixties" throughout society, but also in part to the surprisingly rapid success that gay and lesbian people had in establishing a place in society, at least in the large urban centers. By the early 1980s, much of the gay political establishment in places such as New York and San Francisco had become assimilated into the power structures of their city and, to a lesser degree, state governments and had worked on such issues as the passage of antidiscrimination laws and the establishment of domestic partnership structures. These political insiders were important in enabling groups such as GMHC to forge connections to public health agencies and to garner government funding, but adopted the nonconfrontational, incrementalist tactics that had served them well before the advent of AIDS.[22]

Some of the first coordinated AIDS activism was organized by the media-oriented Gay and Lesbian Alliance Against Defamation (GLAAD), which grew out of an organized demonstration against the homophobic and AIDS-phobic coverage of the *New York Post*. It seemed at first that GLAAD would assume leadership of a new AIDS movement, but the more radically minded were soon disillusioned with the mainstream tactics and hierarchical organization of the new group. "It was pretty tame, as far as I was concerned, and very much in the image of earlier kinds of generally progressive organizations. There was already a board. They already had an idea what they were doing and, basically, they wanted an army of soldiers," noted Maxine Wolfe. Wolfe was also disappointed with the cautious tactics of what she called GLAAD's "very orchestrated demonstrations. By 'orchestrated' I mean they negotiated with the cops, they basically told you when to show up, when to go home, and there was absolutely no input from anybody into what was going to be done."[23]

Partly in reaction to the perceived timidity of the GLAAD agenda, a new gay rights group called the Lavender Hill Mob carried out zaps, or short, disruptive verbal attacks, on the New York City Council, demanding stronger legal protections for people with AIDS facing eviction from their homes. Later, the mob would travel to Atlanta to protest at the headquarters of the Centers for Disease Control and Prevention (CDC), unfurling the banner "TEST DRUGS, NOT PEOPLE" to promote faster approval of anti-HIV drugs and resist mandatory testing for HIV. They identified cumbersome bureaucratic procedures, particularly in clinical drug trials, that slowed the testing and approval of new drugs. They criticized a hidebound scientific establishment that remained inflexibly committed to slow and methodical research policies and procedures even as people were dying around them. And they argued for using the power of the government to promote the welfare of people with HIV rather than to punish or marginalize them.[24]

With their emphasis on these areas, the Lavender Hill Mob presaged the types of drug development issues that would later become central to AIDS treatment activism, yet their particular confrontation with power would prove to be short-lived, and the group shortly thereafter disbanded. Overall, AIDS activism in the early to mid-1980s remained of a fairly mild and diffuse variety. This is not to say that many people who were combating AIDS did not see themselves as being "activist," at least insofar as they were taking active measures to promote health and to combat disease. Many health practitioners, public policy experts, psychologists, academics, service providers, and other professionals radically reoriented their work in the early 1980s to face the new medical, psychosocial, and support needs raised by the spread of the epidemic. Indeed, it is meaningful to speak of such professionals, as well as many committed volunteers, as partially forming what has been alternatively termed an "AIDS community" and "AIDS culture" or even an "AIDS movement."

The impact of this larger response to the challenges posed by AIDS should not be underestimated. Early AIDS professionals and volunteers worked to safeguard privacy rights, dispel myths and misconceptions about HIV transmission, reduce stigma, promote HIV prevention, train professionals to meet the challenges of the epidemic, and underscore the need for compassion and empathy for people with AIDS. Most of this work would not, however, be considered political activism per se, insofar as it was conducted in cooperation with—rather than confrontation with—existing institutions and processes. That would change in 1987.

THE TURN TO ACTIVISM

Six years into the AIDS epidemic, the general population had finally begun to pay attention—but not in the ways that most activists had hoped. The 1985 death of film icon Rock Hudson, who was gay but had long been viewed as the quintessentially heterosexual leading man, had awoken the mass public to the pervasive dangers of AIDS. Yet rather than reflecting sympathy or support, public opinion polls revealed a skyrocketing of homophobic and AIDS-phobic attitudes. HIV-positive children were expelled from their schools after noisy protests by parents, and people with AIDS lost their jobs, homes, and savings even as their partners, friends, and neighbors were falling ill and dying all around them. Right-wing pundits had called for the visible tattooing of people with AIDS, and a California ballot initiative to require the mass quarantining of the HIV-positive had garnered nearly 400,000 signatures. And throughout it all, a pervasive silence emanated from the nation's leader—six years into his presidency, Ronald Reagan had yet to make a public address on the crisis.

At the same time, there was an increasing impulse toward breaking the silence around AIDS, one driven by a concern that the epidemic was no longer confined to marginal—and expendable—high-risk groups but now threatened the more important "general population." With this waning of mass denial and avoidance of AIDS, there emerged a greater sense of urgency about confronting the crisis, opening a window of political opportunity for change. What was unclear was whether the moment would most effectively be seized by those seeking to use the coercive power of the state to treat people with HIV as criminals or those who wanted to use the authority of the state and the vitality of civil society to fight the epidemic itself.

Deeply conservative forces were clearly ascendant in the 1980s, a fact driven home by the shockingly retrograde ruling of the Supreme Court in the case of *Bowers v. Hardwick* in 1986. For over two decades, federal courts had been steadily expanding personal privacy rights, on the basis of the Fourth Amendment and other Constitutional provisions, in such sexuality-related areas as the right to use contraception and the right to terminate a pregnancy. In the *Hardwick* case, police had lawfully entered a Georgia man's home for other purposes and then witnessed him having consensual sex with another man. Michael Hardwick was subsequently prosecuted and convicted under the state's seldom enforced antisodomy laws. Not only did the Supreme Court uphold the Georgia ruling and refuse to extend personal privacy rights to same-sex behavior, but they took the opportunity to heap scorn up upon gay men and lesbians. Any claim to a fundamental right to "commit homosexual sodomy" was "at best facetious" wrote the Court majority, citing the "very ancient roots" of antigay attitudes. Seemingly abandoning Constitutional analysis, Chief Justice Warren Burger wrote that sodomy had been "subject to state intervention throughout the history of Western civilization" and, eschewing the separation of church and state, added that "condemnation of those practices is firmly rooted in Judaeo-Christian moral and ethical standards." Sexual behavior between two members of the same sex, then, was not to be considered a natural expression of intimacy between some members of American society, but a sex crime more akin to rape, child molestation, or bestiality.[25]

On its face, the *Hardwick* decision was almost the reverse of the Supreme Court's ruling in *Brown v. Board of Education*, which had struck down racial segregation and thus the second-class citizenship of African Americans. By denying protection to a defining characteristic of homosexuality, the Supreme Court was not dispelling but reinforcing the criminalized status of gay men and lesbians at the very same time that the community desperately needed the support of government and the protections of its civil liberties. Yet ironically, the *Hardwick* ruling had a galvanizing effect similar to that of *Brown,* contributing to the "cognitive liberation" of an aggrieved population. Whereas *Brown* stoked collective action by demonstrating that African Americans had an ally in the Supreme Court, *Hardwick* awakened gay communities to the fact that they did *not* have such an ally. In the language of social movement theory, southern blacks responded to an "opportunity" while gay communities to "threat"—opposite sides of the same coin.

Already faced with a hostile president, an inertial bureaucracy, a docile Congress, and often complacent city and state government, gay and lesbian communities became aware with a sudden shock that the courts could also not be counted upon to protect their basic civil liberties, much less to expedite a more effective response to AIDS. Compulsory testing and mass quarantines seemed to be that much closer, while a vigorous and coordinated government response to AIDS seemed as far away as ever. Thus the ruling clearly demonstrated that any change to the status quo would have to come as a result of gay and lesbian people's own actions in confrontation with the structures of power. As political scientist and ACT UP member Deborah Gould explained, "In the wake of the Court's ruling, anger among lesbians and gay men became pronounced, evident in op-ed columns and letters-to-the-editor in cities around the country, where it was explicitly linked to the need for 'active resistance,' 'riots,' 'protest,' law-breaking,' 'boycotts,' another 'Stonewall,' a 'return to the streets' . . . a transformation that opened up a space for lesbians and gay men to engage in militant political activism." Gould continued: "By exposing the state's willingness, even eagerness, to exclude an entire class of people from constitutional protections, the *Hardwick* ruling encouraged a more politicized analysis of the government's response to AIDS that precluded any reduction of the epidemic to a tragic string of individual deaths and to isolated feelings of grief."[26]

THE BIRTH OF ACT UP

Amidst this ferment, Larry Kramer gave a historic speech in early March 1987 at the Lesbian and Gay Community Services Center in New York's Greenwich Village. In his speech, Kramer caught the attention of the audience by declaring that most of them might be dead in five years, and then asked a simple pointed question: "Do we want to start a new organization devoted solely to political action?" Where Kramer's earlier calls had failed to unleash "cognitive liberation," this time the answer would prove to be a resounding "yes!" in part because the audience were already primed for action—steeped in grief, living in fear, and feeling abandoned by their government.

"The people who came to the first meeting of ACT UP included individuals from GMHC who had become totally disaffected by its unwillingness to do any political stuff. There were people from the PWA Coalition who wanted to get out on the streets," said Wolfe. At the end of the speech, Kramer asked, "What are we going to do?," and "suddenly, a slight woman in the back stood up and shrieked, 'Act up! Fight back! Fight AIDS,'" recalled eyewitness Maer Roshan. "The entire crowd was on its feet. Next to me, a hollow-cheeked acquaintance struggled up from his wheelchair and joined the chorus, pumped a fist joyfully in the air. He was just thirty, and two months later he was dead. ACT UP, however, lived on."[27]

Kramer's speech and its aftermath had a galvanizing effect similar to that of the Stonewall Riots among a population of sick, dying, frightened, and dispirited people. A few days later, some 300 activists attended the first meeting of the newly founded "AIDS Network," soon to be renamed the AIDS Coalition to Unleash Power, but much more commonly known by the descriptive acronym ACT UP, and had by month's end organized their first action. The flyer for that first action began: "NO MORE BUSINESS AS USUAL!—Come to Wall Street in front of Trinity Church at 7AM Tuesday March 24 for a MASSIVE AIDS DEMONSTRATION" to demand "immediate release by the Federal Food & Drug Administration of drugs that might help save our lives." It concluded: "President Reagan, nobody is in charge! AIDS IS THE BIGGEST KILLER IN NEW YORK CITY OF YOUNG MEN AND WOMEN. Tell your friends. Spread the word. Come protest together . . . AIDS IS EVERYBODY'S BUSINESS NOW." The sponsoring organization was identified as the AIDS Network, "an ad hoc and broad-based community of AIDS-related organizations and individuals."[28]

More particularly, the flyer sketched out the types of goals that would become the mainstay of ACT UP. Much of the focus of the group, and of AIDS treatment activism in general, can be encapsulated in the oft-used slogan "Drugs into Bodies": the goal was to shake loose resources for the development of new drugs, to force them through a sluggish and unresponsive testing process, and to ensure affordable prices. Thus, the flyer called for "immediate abolishment of cruel double-blind studies wherein some get the new drugs and some don't," "immediate release of these drugs to everyone with AIDS," and "immediate availability of these drugs at affordable prices." This compelling need for effective and widely available medications was central to the ACT UP agenda, and would remain so.

Still, the flyer also included other, broader imperatives concerning prevention activism ("immediate massive public education to stop the spread of AIDS") and protection of privacy and other rights ("immediate policy to prohibit discrimination in AIDS treatment, insurance, employment, housing"). And always there was a call for greater governmental leadership and attention ("immediate establishment of a coordinated, comprehensive, and compassionate national policy on AIDS"). Other issues that would become central to the group's focus include the specific needs and rights of women and ethnic/racial minorities, demands for needle-exchange programs and the treatment of drug addiction as a health question rather than a criminal matter, and the securing of access to basic subsistence needs, especially housing.

The inaugural protest on Wall Street set up the confrontational tenor and tone that would become ACT UP's hallmark, as well as several important tactical and organizational precedents. "No permit was sought or provided for the demonstration. Police responded by immediately barricading the picket and limiting its movement. By pre-arranged agreement, however, several volunteers swung into the traffic lanes in an attempt to block cars and trucks from entering Wall Street. The news media was thereby provided with images of 'homosexuals' being handcuffed and dragged into police custody . . . "[29]

That summer at the New York City Gay and Lesbian Pride March, ACT UP captured the imagination of many members of the community with an audacious float traveling down Fifth Avenue. Circled with barbed wire, the float carried people dressed in concentration camp clothing, while members outside, dressed in masks and military gear, handed out flyers and sold ACT UP T-shirts.[30] Subsequently, ACT UP New York meetings would attract as many as 800 people, drawn to the organization's central goal of being a "diverse, non-partisan group united in anger and commitment to direct action to end the AIDS crisis." The meetings were also, to some, the trendy new place to see and be seen—and perhaps to "get laid." ACT UP thus not only drew upon existing linkages, but quickly forged new ones in the heat of battle. "People's entire friendship networks were based in ACT UP," noted Wolfe. "People hadn't felt this connected since the early '70s. And that is a very special moment in an activist history."[31]

Soon, just as in the case of Stonewall, news radiated out from New York, the nation's largest city and its media capital. Then in October 1987, the nascent group had a prime opportunity for national exposure at the second National Lesbian and Gay March on Washington, which placed a heavy emphasis on AIDS and featured the unfolding of the full AIDS Memorial Quilt on the National Mall. ACT UP members distributed to viewers of the quilt a leaflet loaded with the grief and anger that undergirded their activism: "These people have died of a virus. But they have been killed by our government's neglect and inaction. . . . Before this Quilt grows any larger, turn your grief into anger. TURN THE POWER OF THE QUILT INTO ACTION."[32] ACT UP gained even more attention with a raucous demonstration at the offices of the Food and Drug Administration (FDA) involving over 1,000 protestors. This "FDA Action" would become the foundational event of ACT UP at the national level, evidence that the group could spark interest and participation outside of its original home base in Manhattan.[33]

PROLIFERATION

By early 1988, ACT UP chapters had begun to proliferate throughout the United States. In some cases, existing AIDS activist groups, such as Chicago's Dykes and Gay Men Against Repression (DAGMAR) and San Francisco's AIDS Action Pledge, transformed themselves into local chapters of ACT UP. Over time, more than a hundred chapters formed in such U.S. cities as Boston, Los Angeles, Portland (Oregon), Seattle, Houston, and New Orleans, and other chapters on college campuses and in smaller cities also formed, although many were small and short-lived. At the same time, local activists organized ACT UP chapters in such international cities as Sydney, London, Berlin, Amsterdam, Montreal, and Paris; some other groups, notably the Toronto-based AIDS Action Now!, drew inspiration from the ACT UP model without formally assuming the name. The focus of the international chapters was largely on the AIDS crises in their own cities and countries, although there was periodic communication, coordination, and collaboration across borders.

Although ACT UP New York was the first, and in many ways the prototypical and leading, chapter, neither it nor any other body had any central authority over other chapters. The name was deliberately left uncopyrighted, and autonomous new chapters were created simply "when a group of people in a city or region get together and form a group called ACT UP." Although generally rooted principally in preexisting gay and lesbian communities, the new chapters attracted students, nongay PWAs, social justice activists, and many people of general radical leanings. Once a new chapter became established, it could be informally recognized by other chapters if it met "certain qualities that characterize an ACT UP chapter" such as being a democratic, open group committed to direct action as a means of ending the AIDS crisis.[34]

Individual membership was equally informal; as the New York chapter's New Member's Packet states, "You are a member of ACT UP. You became a member by showing up at an ACT UP general meeting, committee meeting, or an action." New members were welcomed to participate in discussions at meetings and to participate in actions, although they were asked to refrain from voting until their third meeting.[35] The commitment to radical democratic practices and full decentralization was pervasive— indeed, the group had no president, no officers, and no paid staff, and all final authority rested with votes from "the floor" of each meeting, with "every member a leader." Although standing committees, including a coordinating committee, were created to facilitate preliminary decision making and administration, they were limited from having the final say so as to avoid "usurping the power and energy residing in the body as a whole."[36]

This commitment to participatory democracy was hugely appealing to many members, but came at a price. Materials produced by ACT UP New York itself conceded that its general meetings "can run very long and become heated and emotional. They can also be tedious and frustrating. It can be extremely confusing and overwhelming for new members and even for old members."[37] Structure came mainly from a meeting order consisting of ninety-second statements announcing activities, "life-saving information" announcements about medical news, presentations on proposed actions and zaps, reports on recent events, and proposals for changes to the internal works of the organization. Linking the group to its base in grief and anger, ACT UP Chicago rejected the idea of opening their meetings with a moment of silence for the dead, replacing it instead with a "moment of rage" marked by a loud chant.[38]

Early group participants were also, in keeping with conventional wisdom, largely white, gay, male, well educated, middle class, and younger. One survey of attendees at ACT UP New York general meetings in mid-1989 revealed a membership that was about 80 percent male; 95 percent lesbian, gay, or bisexual; 90 percent white; 95 percent holders of college or graduate degrees; and 67 percent under age 35.[39] Although white gay men formed the largest contingent of the organization, lesbians and people of color, both men and women, were always deeply involved.

The high level of involvement in ACT UP by lesbians was not a foregone conclusion. Despite the frequent use of the term "gay and lesbian community," homosexual men and women had quite distinct social networks. Politically, lesbians had been more invested in the feminist movement than in the gay male communities formed in city-center "gay ghettos." Further, lesbians had not themselves emerged as a major risk group for HIV infection, in part because female-to-female transmission of HIV is quite rare. Yet many lesbians found in ACT UP a new home for radical politics and direct action that had been missing since the height of the feminist movement in the 1970s. In addition, many of their early efforts were targeted toward protesting the exclusion of women from clinical trials, educating about the risks of HIV to women, and securing the legal and social rights of women, among whom increasing numbers of

HIV and AIDS cases were being diagnosed. In these and other ways, the involvement of lesbian feminists in the AIDS movement represented an extension of their important earlier work around health-related issues such as reproductive rights and general access to quality health care for women.

The position of people of color, especially gay men, was somewhat different insofar as black and Latino men who had sex with men had always been heavily represented among people with HIV. Further, by the late 1980s, nongay segments of communities of color were beginning to be overrepresented among new HIV infections. But the role of people of color in early AIDS activism in some ways reflected the marginalization of black, Latino, and Asian gay men within the larger gay movement, which was often led by white, well-educated, middle-class men seeking assimilation into the larger culture. Insofar as gay men of color were underrepresented in gay professional, social, and neighborhood networks, they initially tended to be underrepresented among activists.

And so fairly early on, ideological splits became evident between more affluent white gay men, who were seen by some as having a narrow agenda concerning drug development and access, and many women and people of color who sought to address broader systemic issues of racism, sexism, homophobia, and class oppression. Sometimes, these tensions could be resolved by broadening the activist agenda through groups such as the ACT UP Women's Caucus, or through loosely affiliated groups such as BAM (Black AIDS Mobilization) and WHAM (Women's Health Action and Mobilization). Yet these tensions also presaged some of the forces that would eventually lead to the fragmentation of the movement in the early 1990s.

TACTICS AND STRATEGIES

Although there were always some disagreements in the priorities afforded to different goals held by ACT UP members, there was a comparatively high level of consensus around questions of tactics and strategies. Indeed, nonviolent direct action was integral to the definition of ACT UP, and those who disagreed with the ACT UP model either did not join the group or did not stay with it.

ACT UP tactics were broadly divided into two categories: quick, nearly spontaneous "zaps" and larger-scale, planned "actions." Zaps were designed "to address AIDS issues needing immediate action by ACT UP. Zaps are a method for ACT UP members to register their disapproval and anger toward the zap target" through such techniques as mass mailings and faxes, picketing, invading offices, distributing fact sheets, and phone

calls. Although on a smaller scale than mass actions, the number of participants still counted: as one ACT UP document stated "the more zappers
who zap the zappee the better the zap."[40]

In contrast, actions were defined as "public protests or demonstrations
organized by a working group within ACT UP. Actions specifically target a
person or organization who is not responding effectively, or morally, to the
AIDS crisis." Actions seek to make specific demands, increase public
awareness, concern, and knowledge, and to submit actions of the target
to media scrutiny, and usually involve a planning period of at least two
weeks, mass promotion, and large-scale participation.[41]

A consistently unifying characteristic among disparate actions and zaps
was a commitment to nonviolent civil disobedience (or CD). ACT UP
New York described CD as "a traditional method of drawing attention to a
cause that was used by members of the American Revolution, Gandhi, and
Rosa Parks to name a few. CD involves breaking a law to draw attention to
a larger injustice in society. People in ACT UP who choose to participate in
CD take responsibility for their decision to risk arrest."[42] Although civil
disobedience led to arrests that tended to provoke the media coverage that
the group sought, some ACT UP members were ambivalent toward being
arrested, with its attendant legal complications, possibility of abuse by police
or prisoners, and other risks. "I never go to a demonstration to get arrested;
I go to demonstrations to bring about change, and am willing to risk arrest
to produce that desired change," wrote member Aldyn McKean. "Getting
arrested is of little significance in and of itself. We're not out to accumulate
arrests like merit badges. Arrests result from our commitment to achieve
change; they are the means to an end, not the end in themselves."[43]

Far from being a spontaneous act of rebellion, then, successful use of CD
required careful planning and structure, including making a list of specific
demands, targeting individuals or groups with the power to meet those
demands, and making the cost of resistance higher than the cost of giving
in. This could be done by creating persistent problems such as occupying an
office or zapping faxes, and by educating the public "in ways that cause
embarrassment to those in power and cause them to be fearful that the
popular movement for change may grow strong enough to threaten
their power."[44] The resolve of many protestors to risk arrest was stiffened
by their knowledge that other group members would be aware of their
whereabouts, trace them through the correctional system, quickly post bail,
and provide them with legal representation.

The group members instinctively understood that the best way to
amplify the message of an action was through the use of visual strategies
that would be particularly striking on television or in photos, and through

the use of striking slogans and pithy aphorisms. It helped enormously that so many members of ACT UP had backgrounds in visual arts, graphic design, theater, and other performing arts as well as in writing, editing, and advertising. Speaking of many early ACT UP organizers, veteran activist Maxine Wolfe noted: "They were well aware, any time we did a demo, that there would be TV cameras present and what these cameras would be looking at. We focused on what would stand out, what would show up. This was in a way that no one I ever knew had done before. It was easy to learn stuff. What color do you make banners when you use them at night as opposed to day? And what size does something have to be to show up? How will this move through space? And I think that was very important because in fact that's exactly what caught the media's attention. We did not just picket around the front of a building, which is totally boring; we broke into the building."[45]

Even the name of the group itself was well suited for buttons and logos (the full name, the "AIDS Coalition to Unleash Power," was actually chosen to fit the acronym). Kramer himself was a playwright able to construct a narrative arc to the epidemic, one which at times stretched back to the Stonewall Riots and often even further back to the Holocaust. One of the group's earliest acts was to adopt a striking logo—an pink triangle reminiscent of those that gay men had to wear in Nazi concentration camps—and a simple slogan in uppercase typeface—"SILENCE=DEATH"—connecting not only to silence about AIDS but further back to "the love that dare not speak its name." The activist orientation of the group soon also led to a companion slogan of "ACTION=LIFE." Other memorable images included day-glo colored photos of Ronald Reagan that recalled the scandal of a Republican predecessor with the term "AIDSGATE" and posters of bloody handprints stating that "The Government Has Blood on Its Hands."[46]

Despite such a dramatic emphasis on style, substance was also not lacking. Indeed, part of the empowerment behind ACT UP involved becoming AIDS experts in their own right, often with the assistance and support of public health and other professionals who were their allies. "Over the course of the epidemic, members of the AIDS movement have taught themselves the details of virology, immunology and epidemiology," wrote sociologist Steven Epstein in a wide-ranging study of the ways in which "knowledge" of AIDS has been constructed. "They have criticized scientific research that seemed to be fueled by anti-gay assumptions, defended speculation about alternative theories of AIDS causation, asserted that community-based AIDS organizations have the expertise to define public health constructs such as 'safe sex,' demanded scientific investigation of potentially useful treatments, established a grassroots base of knowledge about treatments, conducted their own 'underground' drug trials, and criticized the methodologies employed in AIDS clinical research."[47]

ACT UP members also refused to comply with traditional notions of deference from lay people to experts or from doctors to patients. "They have established their credibility as people who might legitimately speak in the language of medical science, in particular with regard to the design, conduct, and interpretation of clinical trials used to test the safety and efficacy of AIDS drugs," wrote Epstein. Their impressive command of both scientific fact and bureaucratic procedures enabled many AIDS activists to secure a voice in institutional arrangements through participation on advisory committees and institutional review boards set up by hospitals, pharmaceutical companies, government agencies, community-based organizations, and other key decision-making bodies.[48]

Still, the rational and "cognitive" were not necessarily the only major elements of what made ACT UP so effective. Indeed, the intensity of protests, zaps, demonstrations, and even some meetings was compelling to many participants, particularly those who themselves had HIV/AIDS. Some had a sense that those participating in early ACT UP actions could claim that they were in a historic vanguard. In a speech at an ACT UP demonstration in Albany, New York, activist Vito Russo said, "AIDS is a real test of us, as a people. When future generations ask what we did in this crisis, we're going to have to tell them that we were out here today. And we have to leave the legacy to those generations of people who will come after us."[49]

Others saw AIDS activism in almost psychotherapeutic terms. "People with AIDS have a lot of things to be afraid of. They may be afraid of rejection, of legal reprisal, of losing their health care, of not being able to work, of losing their jobs, of social rejection. Often, after working through these various fears one uncovers a fear of one's own anger and a fear of one's own power," wrote ACT UP member Jon Greenberg. "ACT UP is an extraordinarily effective tool for people to use to help them confront and get to the other side of their fears."

Greenberg continued: "An ACT UP demonstration with arrests gives people the opportunity to confront and work through their fear of authority. . . . Additionally, and equally important to the process of empowerment, an ACT UP demonstration gives people the opportunity to work out their anger in a public forum so that the anger doesn't continue to hold them back, make them ill, confuse their thinking. . . . ACT UP demonstrations are primal scream therapy for people who would never voluntarily engage in primal scream therapy."[50] Anger and rage had a major place in the lexicon of ACT UP, counterweights to the fear and grief that define the lives of so many people with AIDS.

A LEGACY OF ACCOMPLISHMENT

ACT UP's activity occurred on many levels, ranging from "the floor" of rowdy general meetings to the quieter work of editing videotape of demonstrations and compiling oral histories to the intensive study that made ACT UP members into "lay experts" in their own right. But the group will always be defined by and remembered for its spectacularly choreographed direct actions. Among the most prominent of these between 1987 and 1993 were:

- a "No to *Cosmo*" picket of *Cosmopolitan* magazine by the ACT UP New York Women's Caucus for downplaying the risk of HIV to heterosexual women, which later formed the basis for a documentary film;[51]
- an "alternative freshman orientation" by ACT UP Boston for incoming students at Harvard Medical School, urging them to "challenge the notion of scientists that subjects in research have no rights and may not actively participate in decisions about treatment";[52]
- a take-over of the U.S. headquarters of the transnational pharmaceutical giant Burroughs-Wellcome, during which four ACT UP members used steel plates and rivets to seal themselves in the company's executive offices for eighteen hours, until authorities arrived with blowtorches;[53]
- the shutting-down of trading on the floor of the New York Stock Exchange, with members chained to the VIP balcony using foghorns and a banner to protest the pricing policies of Burroughs-Wellcome (which cut prices for the drug AZT by 20 percent four days later);[54]
- street protests by ACT UP Milwaukee after a seriously ill local man with AIDS was arrested for a traffic violation and kept for forty-eight hours in Racine County Jail, dying several days later;[55]
- a "die-in" on the road to President George H. W. Bush's vacation home in Kennebunkport, Maine, including the unscrolling of a fifty-foot banner outlining a plan to end the AIDS crisis;[56]
- the storming of the 1992 Republican National Convention in Houston by over 2000 protestors, including the burning of an effigy of George H. W. Bush and a chaotic clash with police;[57]
- a "Day of Desperation" that included the invasion of a CBS Evening News program while it was being broadcast, the delivery of coffins to various government officials, and the hanging of a banner over the

arrivals board at New York's Grand Central Station reading "One AIDS Death Every Minute";[58]

- a march on the capital building and governor's mansion in San Juan, Puerto Rico, to protest the lack of treatment for PWAs and failures in prevention efforts;[59]
- protests at the Centers for Disease Control and Prevention (CDC) and the National Institute of Health (NIH) to call for the expansion of the list of AIDS-defining illnesses to include conditions more common among women and people of color and for more inclusion in clinical trials for these populations;[60]
- a highly controversial "Stop the Church" protest of more than 4,500 at St. Patrick's Cathedral against Catholic opposition to condom distribution and safer sex education, during which several demonstrators entered the cathedral itself and one trampled on a communion wafer;[61] and
- several "political funerals" of people who had died of AIDS, including an "Ashes Action" during which cremated remains were scattered on the lawn of the White House.[62]

Taken as a whole, these direct actions were defined by the belief that if silence equaled death, then it followed that action equaled life—the preservation and enhancement of which was the fundamental goal of the AIDS treatment activism of the late 1980s and early 1990s. In all, the list of accomplishments by ACT UP and its allies during their heyday between 1987 and 1993 was impressive. In a comprehensive review, sociologist Steven Epstein identified the following key accomplishments:[63]

- widespread publication in scientific journals and presentations at scientific conferences, which "created new pathways for the dissemination of medical information" and exerted pressure leading to faster release of findings from prestigious journals to the press;
- influence over entrenched practices in drug trials, including which studies would be funded, the number and demographic diversity of those enrolled in drug trails, how soon new drugs would be become available through such mechanisms as expanded access and accelerated approval, and how quickly drugs would move through the approval process;
- securing the use of clinical markers such as CD4 cell counts as important prognostic tools and to expand the definition of AIDS; and
- shifting the balance of power in the doctor-patient relationship by encouraging "health consumers" to be well informed and to challenge their physicians' advice, in the process inspiring other groups such as

people with breast cancer, Alzheimer's disease, chronic fatigue syndrome, and other conditions.

MOVEMENT DECLINE

Despite this impressive list of accomplishments, ACT UP in its heyday was never able to accomplish its one most cherished goal: the development of a cure—the "Holy Grail" of AIDS treatment activism—or even an effective treatment for HIV infection. In fact, by 1993, when the group's major actions and accomplishments were already behind it, the prospects of HIV treatments seemed as remote as ever. In June of that year, results were released from the Concorde Study, a European research initiative to determine the effectiveness of AZT, the first major anti–HIV drug. Activists and people with HIV in general were deeply disheartened when the study revealed that AZT was of very limited value for a limited time, not sub-stantially slowing progression to AIDS or death after an AIDS diagnosis.[64] To many, it felt that not a single step had been taken forward on the treatment front during the dozen years of the epidemic.

The mood of the moment was captured in a *New York Times* editorial entitled "The Unyielding AIDS Epidemic."[65] "No scientific breakthrough is apt to wipe this scourge from the earth any time soon. Indeed, the existing medical weapons against AIDS are less successful than once believed. There is little choice now but to shift the emphasis to prevention programs. . . . What a letdown to find, after a decade of rapid progress in understanding AIDS, that practical medical accomplishments are still years away." The *Times*'s chief medical correspondent, Lawrence K. Altman, wrote, "It is one of the bleakest moments in the fight against the disease since it was first recognized as a new disease in 1981."[66]

And so this was clearly not a moment at which ACT UP could "declare victory" and end their work; yet by this point the group had already peaked and was on the brink of a precipitous decline. This timing, then, suggests that ACT UP's decline cannot be explained in the way that, say, the civil rights movement's decline can be attributed to the achievement of certain crucial goals, such as legislation to mandate desegregation and to enforce voting rights. Yet another common explanation for the decline of social movements—resistance and countermobilization by the movement's oppo-nents—also does not fully explain the decline of ACT UP. Although phar-maceutical companies and their lobbies were constantly evolving strategies to repel activist demands, they usually ended up on the losing side of their confrontations. Likewise, some hidebound and inertial governmental institutions managed to delay or resist the demands of activists. But overall, although many people remained uneasy at the brazen and confrontational tactics used by ACT UP, few could argue with the basic goal of promoting effective treatments for HIV. Thus AIDS activists never encountered truly intense countermobilization such as that faced by, say, civil rights activists or antiwar demonstrators in the 1960s.

In the end, the AIDS treatment movement had few "natural enemies"; *everyone* in society stood to benefit from the more effective treatment of HIV or at least from streamlined and more efficient drug testing and pro-duction methods. Although pitched battles were being fought over issues such as condom distribution, testing laws, and needle exchange in the area of HIV *prevention,* more effective and accessible *treatments* were a goal that could be near-universally shared. Indeed, there was even a love-hate sym-biosis between the pharmaceutical companies and people with HIV, with each side both needing and fearing the other, either as the main producers or consumers of medications. Once government AIDS Drug Assistance Programs (ADAPs) were created in 1990 to provide wide-ranging access to medications, even tensions over domestic pricing became less acute.

Thus the answer to the question of why ACT UP began to decline after 1993 cannot be answered with reference to outside developments but must be explained by way of the movement's internal dynamics and character-istics of its membership. In the absence of any effective treatment for HIV infection, many members found themselves leapfrogging from one unpro-mising clinical trial to another, all the while seeing their own t-cell counts decline. Some stayed healthy but burned out psychologically and withdrew from activism. Others returned to their roots in non-AIDS-centered gay and lesbian activism, such as those who founded the influential, if short-lived, radical group Queer Nation, which became famous for same-sex "kiss ins" at suburban malls and the slogan "We're Here. We're Queer. Get Used to It."[67] With the success of prevention campaigns, fewer gay men were becoming HIV-infected and the center of gravity in the gay community began to shift to new issues. Where the focus of the 1987 Gay and Lesbian March on Washington was squarely on AIDS, the 1993 march emphasized issues such as the service of gay people in the military and the fight for same-sex marriage.[68]

Still other people moved away from the more confrontational tactics of ACT UP toward more conventional action. In 1992, a number of core ACT UP members broke off to form the Treatment Action Group (TAG), which broke with a number of foundational ACT UP policies by establishing invitation-only memberships (which could be revoked by the board), having a paid staff, and accepting donations from pharmaceutical companies. This provoked "considerable criticism from some ACT UP members and other activists. Because the organization is perceived by some as small, elitist, and undemocratic, it has been attacked for not fully representing the interests of the larger AIDS activist movement."[69] Other activists moved into narrower subfields, forming such radical but more specialized groups as Housing Works and the HIV Law Project. These refocused operations in many ways continued to carry the militant mantle but abandoned ACT UP's steadfast refusal to hire paid staff or to engage the government through legal channels.

Perhaps the most controversial splintering occurred when ACT UP San Francisco was taken over by individuals who aligned themselves with "denialists," who claim that HIV is not the cause of AIDS and that therefore any attention paid to HIV prevention was misplaced, wasteful, and ultimately homophobic. In a bizarre twist, this denialist group soon made common cause with AIDS-phobic right-wingers, who also sought to divert attention and funding away from the epidemic by claiming that the disease was self-inflicted and that scarce funds would be better spent on other health needs. Longtime AIDS activists were enraged, but because of ACT UP's radical decentralization and lack of authoritative leadership structures, there was no way to prevent the collapse of what had been one of the nation's preeminent ACT UP chapters. Some longtime ACT UP members formed a new, and more authentic, chapter which at first called itself ACT UP Golden Gate but eventually switched to Survive AIDS so as to avoid the taint of association with the denialist group.[70]

Although much important work continued both within the ACT UP framework and within its offshoots, a sense of gloom settled in on the movement as progress against HIV—much less a cure—remained out of reach. As was so often the case, the mood of burnout was presciently captured as early as 1990 by Larry Kramer, when he wrote, "It is beyond comprehension why, in a presumably civilized country, in the modern era, such a continuing, extraordinary destruction of life, is being attended to so tentatively, so meekly, and in such a cowardly fashion. The armies of the infected, their families, loved ones, and friends no longer know how to deliver their pleas for help. Every conceivable method has been attempted, from quietly working from within to noisily demonstrating without."[71]

All of these factors—burnout and deaths, organizational splintering, and a pervasive sense of hopelessness—were present on election day 1992, the day that ACT UP would lose their prime antagonists and the focus of their anger: the conservative Republican administrations of Ronald Reagan and George H. W. Bush. By comparison, Democratic candidate Bill Clinton said many of the things that AIDS activists wanted to hear, and adopted a far more conciliatory tone. This was especially so on April 2, 1992, when he was publicly confronted by ACT UP member Rob Rafsky at a New York City fundraiser. In the widely broadcast exchange, Clinton asked what he should be doing to demonstrate his commitment to AIDS, then two days later met with members of ACT UP and the group United for AIDS Action (UAA). He agreed to give a major AIDS policy address, to have HIV-positive speakers at the Democratic National Convention, and signed on to the UAA's five-point plan.[72] On October 11, 1992, ACT UP members scattered the ashes of people who had died of AIDS on the front lawn of the White House; less than a month later they were widely rejoicing at the end of the Reagan–Bush era[73] (unaware at the time that Clinton's tenure would come to include many disappointments for AIDS activists, particularly in the area of HIV prevention).

The disintegration of a once-vocal activist community was reflected in a powerful cover story by reporter Jeffrey Schmalz in *The New York Times Magazine* on November 28, 1993. Schmalz wrote that "the AIDS movement was built on grassroots efforts. Now those efforts are in disarray. Many ACT UP leaders have died. The group's very existence was based on the belief that AIDS could be cured quickly if only enough money and effort were thrown at it—something that now seems increasingly in doubt. Besides, it is hard to maintain attacks against a government that is seeking big increases in AIDS spending. Much of the cream of ACT UP has fled, forming groups like TAG and joining mainstream AIDS organizations like Gay Men's Health Crisis and the American Foundation for AIDS Research."[74] Poignantly, Schmalz died of AIDS just two days after the publication of his article. Acutely aware of his own impending death, he ended his article with a *cri de coeur* that reflected the frustration of so many: "There is a phrase that I want shouted at my funeral and written on the memorial cards, a phrase that captures the mix of cynicism and despair that I feel right now and that I will almost certainly take to my grave: *Whatever happened to AIDS?*"

And yet despite its virtual disintegration, ACT UP never did disappear entirely. Its dormant networks sprang back into life episodically, its members continued to deploy their organizational skills in other settings, the group's influence on the public health and biomedical establishments remained in place. And a few chapters even managed to retain at least an organizational shell—which would be available for reactivation a few years later when effective treatments at last became available for the wealthy nations of the world even as the poorer nations were excluded. This second act in the life of ACT UP, as part of a broader coalition of global AIDS treatment activists, is the subject of the next chapter.

Chapter 2

Bridging the Gap: Mobilizing a Global Response

A gloomy mood prevailed as the fifteenth anniversary of the emergence of the epidemic passed on June 5, 1996. In the developed world, the death toll had mounted steadily, with many of those infected in the early to mid-1980s falling sick and dying throughout the early to mid-1990s. A depressingly predictable cycle had developed in which promising new treatments were heralded based on lab experiments only to prove disappointing in clinical terms. Subsequent academic studies would then confirm what doctors and patients alike already knew: that HIV mutated much too quickly for any one drug or any combination of chemically similar drugs to be of much use. In 1994, the organizers of the International AIDS Conference decided to switch to a biannual schedule, since the slow pace of advances could no longer justify a yearly meeting.

As the leading figures in AIDS research and medicine prepared to fly to Vancouver, British Columbia, for the 11th International AIDS Conference in July 1996, however, there was a hopeful buzz in the air. Early reports indicated that experimental protease inhibitors, when used in combination with other antiretroviral medications, had proven highly effective in halting the immune damage wrought by HIV. But it was not until a series of reports revealed the true extent of the power of combination therapies that it appeared that AIDS treatment was about to be revolutionized. It was this major scientific breakthrough that shortly would combine with two other broad socioeconomic processes—the explosion of AIDS in the developing world and the growth of processes of globalization—to set the stage for the emergence of a new AIDS treatment activist movement focused on the developing world.

THE SEARCH FOR TREATMENTS

Before 1996, the struggle to find effective treatment methods to cripple HIV or to undo its damage by boosting the immune system had been painfully slow, even for long stretches of time seemingly at a standstill. This was particularly true coming after several early successes, notably the discovery of HIV in 1983 and the licensing of a test for HIV antibodies in 1985. From a clinical perspective, these two steps were especially significant because they enabled the diagnosis of HIV infection before it progresses to end-stage illness; indeed, antibodies to HIV are usually detectable within the first few weeks of infection. Because the earliest people with AIDS often did not get medical care until they had immune damage that was extensive and illnesses that were severe, they usually died quickly. Earlier identification of HIV infection made it possible to try to at least postpone the onset of serious medical illness.

One early therapeutic strategy against AIDS involved attempts to boost the immune system, an approach that made intuitive sense but failed to yield very useful results, sometimes slipping more into "New Age-ish" wishful thinking than quantifiable medical outcomes. More promising, if still limited, were efforts to prevent or mitigate the more than two dozen conditions identified as "AIDS-defining illnesses." Since many of the first AIDS deaths came from *Pneumocystis carinii* pneumonia, special focus was placed on prophylactic treatments such as inhalation of aerosolized pentamidine or use of the powerful antibiotic Bactrim to prevent the illness. Prophylactic treatment for PCP turned out to be a major success, but other diseases proved harder to forestall, especially as the disease progressed. And, most important, the development of effective treatments for HIV infection itself proved incredibly elusive.

Once HIV had been isolated and studied, it also became possible by the mid-1980s to develop pharmacological weapons that attacked the replication of the virus itself rather than just the diseases that resulted from the compromise of the immune system. Whereas most viruses retain their genetic information on strands of DNA, retroviruses such as HIV employ simpler RNA. The virus's outer coat consists of particular glycoproteins, which can form biochemical bonds with specific proteins (particularly one known as CD4) that are found on the surface of some cells, notably those in the immune system. Once bonding occurs, the HIV life cycle requires the insertion of its own genetic material into the host cell and, ultimately, the use of three important viral enzymes. The first, reverse transcriptase, converts RNA into DNA (a process called "reverse transcription"). The second, integrase, integrates the DNA into the human cell's DNA. The third, protease, later cleaves off new copies of the viral proteins, allowing new virus particles to be assembled and enabling these new viruses to leave the cell.[1]

In 1986, the U.S. Food and Drug Administration (FDA) approved the first antiretroviral drug, AZT (also called zidovudine or Retrovir), for use in preventing HIV replication by inhibiting the activity of the reverse transcriptase enzyme. AZT is part of a class of drugs formally known as nucleoside analog reverse transcriptase inhibitors (RTIs). Over time, several other nucleoside drugs were added to the anti-HIV arsenal, as were a class of nonnucleoside RTIs which work in similar ways to nucleosides but which are more quickly activated once inside the bloodstream. Despite this proliferation of drug options, the standard antiretroviral therapy for HIV-infected individuals between 1986 and 1995 for the most part remained "monotherapy," or treatment with a single drug. Such drugs appeared to be partly efficacious, although there was a great deal of variation in effectiveness among individuals.[2]

During this period, there were also significant advances in the understanding of how HIV functions in the body. The belief that individuals went into a period of "clinical latency" of ten years or more after their initial infection with HIV was replaced with an understanding that huge amounts of viral replication continued throughout the entire period of infection, even if an individual was not exhibiting any symptoms of illness. Thus, the onset of symptoms of AIDS came to be recognized as the result not of a sudden resurgence of a latent virus, but rather of a slow "war of attrition" between HIV and the host immune system, with the latter slowly being whittled away by the former.[3]

The recognition of the persistence of viral replication—with billions of copies of HIV being produced and destroyed daily—also made possible a better understanding of the process by which the virus gradually becomes less sensitive to specific antiretroviral medications, a process known as "developing resistance." Such resistance generally occurs when a random mutation during the replication of HIV causes a small genetic change in the virus's RNA, in the process making it less vulnerable to the effects of antiretroviral drugs. Drug resistance can seriously complicate treatment by rendering drugs less effective or even completely ineffective. Further, once an organism has developed resistance to one drug, it can also become resistant to other drugs in the same class ("cross-resistance") or to a number of different drugs ("multiple-drug resistance"). From this perspective, it could be seen that monotherapy against HIV was of limited usefulness because HIV could quickly develop resistance to any one drug and eventually any one class of drugs.[4] But through the 1980s and into the early

1990s, progress on new classes of drugs was stymied. The first human retrovirus had been identified only in 1980 and the field of retrovirology was still in its infancy. Likewise, the then-prevalent standards for clinical drug trials emphasized slow, steady, and unhurried progress, a stance ill-suited for combating a raging epidemic, which made the clinical trial system a lightning rod for protest by ACT UP and others.

The major breakthrough, the one announced at the 1996 International AIDS Conference in Vancouver, finally came with the development of a new class of drugs that operated differently from the existing reverse transcriptase inhibitors by targeting a different enzyme, protease. These protease inhibitors (PIs) operate in ways quite unlike RTIs in that they do not seek to prevent the infection of a host cell but rather to prevent an already infected cell from producing more copies of HIV. PIs alone had a certain degree of efficacy in combating HIV, but they were especially potent when used in combination with RTIs. Switching from monotherapy (treatment with single drugs) to combination therapy (treatment with drugs from two or more classes) had dramatic effects because it prevents the emergence of mutated forms of HIV before they have the opportunity to proliferate. While random mutation might lead to a form of the virus that is naturally resistant to one class of drugs, it is much rarer that a random mutation might confer resistance to two or more drugs. This is particularly the case when at least one drug targets reverse transcriptase and at least one targets protease.[5]

Taken together, the nucleoside RTIs, nonnucleoside RTIs, and PIs came to be known as "highly active antiretroviral therapy" or HAART. Soon after the announcement at the International AIDS Conference announcement at Vancouver in July 1996 of amazing success in suppressing viral replication, the use of so-called triple combination cocktails became the standard of care in the developed world for HIV-positive individuals who had begun to show signs of significant immunosuppression, such as an opportunistic infection or a low CD4 cell count. The impact was overwhelming, with far fewer individuals progressing from HIV infection to "full blown" AIDS, many fewer new cases of new AIDS-related opportunistic infections and cancers, improved health and well-being among those already diagnosed with AIDS, decreased incidence of transmission from mother to child, and, most notable of all, a plummeting death rate. Between 1995 and 1997, AIDS death rates in the United States declined by more than two-thirds, and new AIDS diagnoses were down by 30 percent.[6] On an individual basis, HAART restored so many people to improved health that some referred to a "Lazarus syndrome" in which people were snatched back from the brink of death. Indeed, among many, the amount of HIV in their bloodstream, their "viral load," became undetectable, which is not to say that it was entirely gone but that it had dropped to levels so low that they could not be detected by existing blood tests.

Even while some were touting the "end of the epidemic," it soon became clear that the new treatments did not by any means constitute a "cure." Most notably, early hopes for the "eradication" of HIV—its complete elimination from the body of an infected individual—went unrealized. While HAART is effective in reducing viral load in blood plasma, HIV also directly infects the cells of the central nervous system and other parts of the body that are not readily reached by medications and thus form so-called sanctuary sites. The virus in such cells can remain latent, and thus beyond the reach of antiretroviral drugs that are able to prevent most new replication but not to flush out latent cells. These latent cells can later resurge into the bloodstream when the immune system is stimulated by something as seemingly minor as flu or a small infection.

Another major disappointment was that some people, particularly those who had been living with AIDS for a long period of time, had sustained so much underlying damage that their bodies simply could not recover, leading to a second decline in health after a brief rebound. Yet another barrier is that antiretroviral treatment regimens are often complicated and challenging, requiring multiple doses of different medications on rigid timetables with often competing requirements, such as being taken with or without food, and with short-term side effects such as nausea, vomiting, and diarrhea. Even a few missed or mistaken doses, however, could promote drug resistance and eventual drug failure, leaving individuals once again susceptible to AIDS-related illnesses. Time has also shown that the powerful HAART medications can have more serious longer-term side effects that could undermine quality of life and lead to heart, kidney, liver, and other diseases. Perhaps the most unusual side effect has been lipodystrophy, or the redistribution of body fat from the face and extremities to the back, neck, and stomach, leading to readily recognizable (and increasingly stigmatized) sunken facial features and engorged torsos. Lipodystrophy can also lead to release of lipids into the blood stream, with resultant serious risk of cardiovascular disease and stroke.

Likewise, even as HIV treatments were making dramatic advances, cases of new HIV infections in the United States seemed to be remaining stable. The relationship between treatment and prevention has been somewhat ambiguous. On the one hand, there is evidence that treatments that reduce viral load in the bloodstream also reduce it in semen and vaginal/cervical secretions, making sexual transmission less likely. On the other hand, treatments also appear to have lifted the pall of fear surrounding HIV infection and weakened the commitment to safer sex and safer drug use, particularly among younger people who never experienced the epidemic at its height and for whom HIV is simply a fact of life. Equally troubling is that drug-resistant strains of HIV can be transmitted in the same ways as any other kind, meaning that some newly infected individuals may *start out* with a strain of virus which cannot be treated effectively with currently existing medications. Evidence has also emerged that some HIV-positive individuals can become "superinfected" with new strains of HIV, including ones that are already drug resistant.

All of these are serious issues, which over time dampened the initial euphoria that followed the release of HAART in 1996. Still, the enormous distance between outright despair and guarded hope should not be understated. The introduction of combination antiretroviral therapies represents the single most important shift in the history of the AIDS epidemic—transforming HIV infection from a "death sentence" into a serious but far more manageable chronic illness for many, although not all, of those living with HIV.

Given the lack of a national health program in the United States, it was not inevitable that the scientific breakthroughs that led to the development of antiretroviral medications would for the most part be made available to the broad majority of Americans who needed them. In 1987 after AZT first became available, states developed a $30 million program to help people with AIDS who lacked sufficient health insurance. In 1990, the landmark Ryan White Comprehensive AIDS Resources Emergency (CARE) Act included provisions for AIDS Drug Assistance Programs (ADAPs) as part of its Title II funding to U.S. states and territories.[7]

ADAPs started off slowly, however, because there were relatively few drugs available for the treatment of AIDS. Likewise, at that time, the official definition of clinical AIDS required diagnosis with one of about two dozen AIDS-defining illness in an HIV-positive person. However, under activist pressure, the U.S. Centers for Disease Control and Prevention in 1993 altered the definition of clinical AIDS. Part of the revision was to expand the list of AIDS-defining illnesses to include invasive cervical cancer, a condition unique to women, and pulmonary tuberculosis, which is usually found among injecting drug users. These changes thus promoted the diagnosis of AIDS in two important but undercounted groups. More radical, though, was a revision of the case definition to include any HIV-positive person whose count of CD4 cells (the type of white blood cell destroyed by HIV) fell below the level of 200 per cubic milliliter.[8]

By clearly defining HIV disease in terms of damage to the immune system, a significantly larger number of people with HIV became eligible for support from programs funded by ADAPs. After protease inhibitors were introduced, this precedent proved hugely important, since it meant that large numbers of Americans living with HIV would have access to a broad formulary of antiretroviral drugs. Some heavily impacted populations such as prisoners, undocumented immigrants, and drug users continued to lack adequate health care on many levels, including access to antiretroviral drugs. But overall, ADAP programs were essential in helping to make the promise of combination antiretroviral drugs widely available in the United States.

THE GAP EMERGES

In stark contrast to the major advances and burgeoning hope seen in the developed world, the mid-1990s were a period of catastrophic expansion in the epidemic in the developing world. The spread of AIDS was not immediately recognized in places like sub-Saharan Africa, the Caribbean, and Southeast Asia; indeed, it was all too easy to miss the emergence of yet another deadly disease in regions of the world besieged with multiple health crises and health systems ill-equipped to treat and track them. Further, the spread of AIDS in the "Global South" occurred in different patterns than in the "Global North," most notably in that heterosexual contact was the overwhelming means of transmission, with mother-to-child infections consequently also much more common. Poverty and lack of access to health care meant that Africans with AIDS typically died from different opportunistic infections than people in developed countries, especially tuberculosis or enteric diseases whose effects were frequently exacerbated by malnutrition and other underlying health deficits. It took some time, for instance, before the "slim disease" of Africa was clearly identified as the same "wasting syndrome" found among many PWAs in the West, which occurs when HIV disrupts the gastrointestinal system and leads to the loss of lean body mass.

In part because the impact of AIDS was conflated with, and obscured by, so many other endemic health problems, awareness of the epidemic grew slowly. Resource limitations and weak public health systems offered few opportunities to conduct widescale HIV testing, mount educational campaigns, or carry out surveillance studies of HIV seroprevalence. AIDS was in many ways avoided until it became unavoidable, when not only individuals but entire families and communities began to die in the late 1990s.

"The Human Immunodeficiency Virus (HIV) which causes AIDS has brought about a global epidemic far more extensive than what was predicted even a decade ago," wrote the United Nations Joint Programme on

HIV/AIDS (UNAIDS) in 2000: "UNAIDS and the World Health Organization (WHO) now estimate that the number of people living with HIV or AIDS at the end of the year 2000 stands at 36.1 million. This is more than 50 percent higher than what WHO's Global Program on AIDS projected in 1991 on the basis of the data then available."[9]

This same UN report also clearly indicated a growing concentration of HIV/AIDS cases in the developing world. By 2000, the AIDS crisis was particularly pronounced in sub-Saharan Africa, where overall adult HIV prevalence rates were estimated at 8.8 percent of the adult population, some 25.3 million people. This statistic stood in stark contrast to adult HIV seroprevalence rates 14.6 times lower in North America (0.6 percent of adults, or 920,000 people) and 36.6 times lower in Western Europe (0.24 percent of adults, or 540,000 people).[10] There are also rapidly growing epidemics elsewhere in the developing world, most notably 5.8 million people in South and Southeast Asia (0.56 percent adult seroprevalence), 1.4 million people in Latin America (0.5 percent adult seroprevalence), and 390,000 people in the Caribbean (2.3 percent adult seroprevalence).

Still, the magnitude of the catastrophe in sub-Saharan Africa is thus far unparalleled. "HIV has penetrated every country across the globe. But one continent is far more touched by AIDS than any other. Africa is home to 70% of adults and 80% of the children living with HIV in the world, and has buried three-quarters of the more than 20 million people worldwide who have died of AIDS since the epidemic began. Over and above the personal suffering that accompanies HIV infection wherever it strikes, the virus in Sub-Saharan Africa threatens to devastate whole communities, rolling back decades of progress toward a healthier and more prosperous future."[11]

The shocking impact of AIDS made it clear that the African epidemic was being driven by far more than individual risk behaviors—that its deeper causes lay in contextual factors that made HIV risk likely or even inevitable. Two interrelated variables are particularly salient: economic status and human rights. Throughout the world, marginalized groups and subpopulations have consistently proven to be most vulnerable to HIV infection. In the developing world, those who are denied equal access to basic societal goods such as education, health care, and employment opportunities and those who are not treated equally in legal systems regarding everything from criminal justice to property rights are usually also those with elevated risks of HIV/AIDS. Likewise, dire economic circumstances (often created or accelerated by the denial of rights) create situations where risk behaviors are more likely to occur, and where HIV infection is more likely to occur and progress more rapidly to AIDS.

The dire circumstances created by poverty are particularly salient in sub-Saharan Africa because poverty itself is particularly salient there. The World Bank's 2004 figures list thirty-eight of the forty-eight sub-Saharan African nations as "low income economies," defined as having per capita gross national incomes of $825 per year or less.[12] Of the few nations not listed as "low income," several are small island nations and the few larger nations that appear to have relatively larger gross national incomes are actually masking another severe form of societal poverty—extreme income inequality within the countries. This is particularly true in South Africa and Botswana, and it is not coincidental that both have HIV/AIDS caseloads, in absolute numbers in the first case and relative numbers in the second, unsurpassed by other nations.

This poverty has been further exacerbated by the imposition of structural adjustment programs by international financial institutions, which required indebted nations seeking further loans to cut their own social spending for education, health, and other services and goods. These policies were most strongly felt by those who could least afford the newly imposed user fees for these services. The attendant impacts on general health would further predispose the poor to even greater susceptibility to HIV. As one analysis explained this predisposition, "the old adage—that if it doesn't kill you, it makes you stronger—is unfortunately not true. Recurrent malnutrition, infectious disease, and parasite infestation, if they don't kill you, make you weaker."[13] The cycle set in place by poverty, at the national and the individual level, is thus a truly vicious one: poverty forces decreased expenditures on health, which in turn leads to poor health, which in turn leads to greater susceptibility to HIV. The full extent of this dynamic is the subject of continuing research, but specific connections have been documented. A study published in 2005, for example, demonstrated that HIV-infected people who are coinfected with malaria have significantly increased viral loads, which in turn may lead to enhanced HIV transmission and accelerated disease progression.[14]

In the case of sub-Saharan Africa, the prevalence of poverty and the failure to ensure basic human rights helps to explain why AIDS has taken such a dramatic toll. These factors also help to explain why the spread is most severe among women, especially young women. By 2000, UNAIDS was estimating for sub-Saharan Africa that "12 to 13 women were becoming newly infected for every 10 men."[15] Under the influence of the traditionalist systems of patriarchy that continue to exist in most sub-Saharan societies, women are frequently unable to make most major decisions in their own lives. In places where women (and children) are regarded as more or less the "property" of the husband and his family, decisions about reproduction become the province of these "owners." When women are denied property, inheritance, and other legal rights, they have little say in how and when sex will occur. Thus wives are vulnerable to infection from nonmonogamous husbands even when they themselves remain faithful, young women may be physically or economically coerced into risky sex work, and all women are vulnerable to sexual assault in places where rape laws do not exist or are poorly enforced.

The impact of HIV/AIDS is disproportionate among women and girls, even when they are not themselves infected. When HIV causes sickness in a household there is almost always a concurrent need for more resources (for medicine, nutritious food, and nursing materials) at the same time as there is the loss of the income formerly generated by the sick person. In such situations, women and girls, whose property and autonomy rights are not protected, will disproportionately bear the brunt of household rationing of health care, food, and school fees. In Kenya, for example, one study showed that in the least HIV-affected Eastern Province, 42 percent of grade five primary school students were girls, but in the heavily affected Nyanza Province only 6 percent of children in the same grade were girls.[16] Because of rigid divisions of labor relegating care giving to women and girls, they bear the overwhelming burden of nursing care, child care (including the care of orphans), and food provision in families affected by AIDS. This human cost has been rendered mostly invisible by terms like "voluntarism" and "home health care," but the real cost was noted in a speech by the director of the United Nations Development Fund for Women (UNIFEM), who concluded that "women remain at home, outside the public sphere, excluded from decision-making, deprived of opportunities to become self-reliant, economically independent, full citizens with power and authority over their own lives, and participatory roles in the world they inhabit."[17]

Beyond the misery caused to individuals and families is the impact of HIV/AIDS within whole societies. Indeed, once it reaches a certain level in any given country, AIDS can actually begin to undermine the entire economy. This is because, historically, most diseases have affected the oldest people, small children, or those who were born with birth defects. Of course, societies do—or at least should—value these individuals and try to protect and support them. But societies do not typically rely upon the elderly, the very young, or the infirm to drive their economies; they look, rather, to those in their prime. This is what makes AIDS so insidious and dangerous to economies: it often strikes the very people in their twenties, thirties, and forties upon whom societies rely for productivity. AIDS thus deprives families and societies of the individuals most capable of farming, laboring, or carrying out other types of crucial work—and also prevents them from passing their skills down to younger people. Decades of inter-mittent progress after decolonization are rapidly being reversed across sub-Saharan Africa.

In affluent countries such as the United States or those in Western Europe, where HIV seroprevalence rates are low by global standards and where many people with HIV can work with the aid of antiretroviral therapies, the economic impact of AIDS relates largely to health care expenditures. But in poor countries with heavy HIV caseloads and few treatment options, AIDS can be economically devastating. One stark study of AIDS-affected families in Zambia, for instance, found that "monthly disposable income in more than two-thirds of the families in the study fell by more than eighty percent."[18] Even death itself creates still more hardship because of funeral expenses.

The advent of antiretroviral therapies might have been able to mitigate the most disastrous consequences of HIV in the developed world—but their availability was limited to only the tiniest fraction of HIV-positive people in the global South. In a groundbreaking and hugely influential article about the treatment of HIV in Brazil, journalist Tina Rosenberg summarized the situation: "[T]he triple therapy that has made AIDS a manageable disease in wealthy nations was considered realistic only for those who could afford to pay $10,000 to $15,000 a year or lived in societies that could. The most that poor countries could hope to do was prevent new cases of AIDS through educational programs and condom promotion or to cut mother-to-child transmission and, if they were very lucky, treat some of AIDS's opportunistic infections. But the 32.5 million people with HIV in the developing world had little hope of survival."[19]

GLOBALIZATION AND THE AIDS EPIDEMIC

This stark bifurcation in AIDS treatment access between the developed and developing world was all the more ironic because it was occurring alongside processes that were drawing the planet together in unprecedented ways. The end of the Cold War in the early 1990s eliminated the Iron Curtain and lifted a major barrier to the free flow of people, ideas, and capital. The expansion of the World Wide Web in the mid-1990s collapsed distances and made global information exchange and communication far easier than ever before. And, most of all, the mid-1990s saw the coalescence of new patterns of economic, social, and cultural interaction, processes most commonly called "globalization."

For a word that is so widely used, globalization is a term fraught with ambiguities. One survey of the use of it found that the term has five distinct commonly used meanings, each of which relates to the AIDS epidemic with varying degrees of significance. *Internationalization* refers to "increases in interaction and interdependence between people in different countries." *Universalization* implies the spread of certain phenomena "to all habitable corners of the planet." *Trade liberalization* implies that "a global world is one without regulatory barriers to transfers of resources between countries." *Westernization/Americanization* connotes "a process of homogenization, as all the world becomes western, modern, and more particularly, American." And finally, *supraterritoriality* suggests the "the growth of 'supraterritorial' relations between people [and] ... the proliferation and spread of ... transborder or transworld connections."[20]

All of these meanings of globalization bear upon the AIDS epidemic. For instance, AIDS is *international* in the sense that transmission easily crosses over borders, and is *universal* in the sense that it is a global pandemic. More significantly for present purposes, however, is the sense of globalization as relating to *trade liberalization,* since the concept of free trade was the driving force behind the rise of powerful multinational corporations free to do business anywhere in the world with few barriers or restrictions. Globalization in the sense of *westernization/Americanization* is relevant in the idea that U.S.-defined concepts of intellectual property rights should govern the approaches taken in other countries to address public health emergencies. Finally, globalization as *supraterritoriality* is also relevant in the sense that multinational corporations have become subject to no single national authority, but also in the sense that activists can form coalitions and connections that transcend older "international" connections by largely bypassing the organizing logic of the territorial nation-state.

While globalization remains an inchoate process, its most tangible expressions are in the form of enhanced authority on the part of a number of intergovernmental organizations such as the International Monetary Fund (IMF), the World Bank, and the World Trade Organization (WTO). Founded in 1995 out of the former General Agreement on Tariffs and Trade, the WTO is a particularly formidable expression of globalization. Almost uniquely among multilateral international organizations, the WTO, for instance, is vested with the ability to enforce its rulings, giving it an authority that exceeded that of such organizations as the World Health Organization or even the United Nations itself.[21]

One of the most significant of the multilateral treaties that forms the basis for globalization is the Agreement on Trade-Related Aspects of Intellectual Property Rights, commonly known as TRIPS, which is administered by the WTO and binding on all WTO members. Its Preamble states that TRIPS was created to "reduce distortions and impediments to international trade..., to promote effective and adequate protection of intellectual property rights, and to ensure that measures and procedures to enforce intellectual property rights do not themselves become barriers to legitimate trade."[22] The TRIPS framework was first developed by a twelve-member ad hoc Intellectual Property Committee, in cooperation with representatives from major industrialized countries, to codify and then extend the patent, copyright, trademark and other forms of protection that then existed for such types of intellectual property as pharmaceuticals, software, and recorded entertainment.[23] Essentially, the major industries wrote the very regulations that were meant to govern them.

"TRIPS is a dramatic expansion of the rights of IP owners and a significant instance of the exercise of private power. The approach embodied in the TRIPS Agreement, extending property rights and requiring high levels of protection, represents a significant victory for U.S. private sector activists from knowledge-based industries. In the TRIPS case, private actors worked together, exercised their authority and achieve a result that effectively narrows the options open to sovereign states and firms, and extends the opportunities of those firms that succeeded in gaining multilateral support for a tough global IP instrument."[24] One reason that the TRIPS framework is viewed as enormously powerful is its placement under the WTO aegis, which means that violations of the treaty are punishable via trade sanctions or other mechanisms both by the WTO and by actions taken by the government of any large economy, most notably the United States.

Among the most controversial areas of contention regarding TRIPS has been its provisions covering access to pharmaceuticals, which had not previously been subject to such high levels of patent protection. Although many areas of intellectual property may have implications for human health and well-being, the question of access to life-enhancing and even lifesaving drugs is uniquely significant. In what was regarded as a loss by the pharmaceutical industry, Article 30 of TRIPS states that "members may provide limited exceptions to the exclusive rights conferred by a patent." Article 31, Section B provides guidelines for the use of intellectual property without authorization of the right holder, but includes the clause that parts of the guidelines "may be waived by a Member in the case of a national emergency or other circumstances of extreme urgency or in cases of public non-commercial use."[25]

This provision was widely seen as applying clearly to the case of pharmaceutical patents, a case made by multiple agencies including the European nongovernmental organizations Médecins San Frontières (Doctors Without Borders) and Health Action International, and the U.S.-based

Consumer Project on Technology. These and other advocates, as well as international organizations such as the World Health Assembly, advanced two approaches in particular, both of which had been included within the TRIPS framework as last resorts for exactly the sort of health catastrophes being created by AIDS. The first approach, *parallel importing,* exploits the fact that for a variety of market-based and regulatory reasons, the same drug may be priced at very different levels in different countries. Parallel importing results when governments allow the importation not only of drugs at the prices set by pharmaceutical companies for any specific country, but also from other countries which pay much lower prices established through policies set by their governments.[26]

The second approach, however, was even more promising: *compulsory licensing,* which would allow countries to authorize the manufacture of generic versions of drugs without the permission of the patent holder as long as they paid a "reasonable royalty."[27] Such a process would dramatically lower the per-unit cost of drugs, since the cost of manufacture is generally only a small fraction of the price charged by pharmaceutical companies, who claim that their drastic price mark-ups are needed to recoup their expenditures in drug research and development. Despite denial on the part of the pharmaceutical companies, however, it was becoming increasingly clear to activists that the prices of many drugs bore no particular relationship to their actual cost of development and production. As Arnold S. Relman and Marcia Angell, two former editors of the *New England Journal of Medicine,* wrote: "[R]esearch and development (R&D) constitutes only a relatively small part of the budgets of the large drug companies. Their marketing and advertising expenditures are much greater than their investment in R&D. Furthermore, they make more in profits than they spend on R&D. In fact, their profits are consistently much higher than those of any other American industry." They noted further that much of the costly preliminary research into many drugs is conducted not by pharmaceutical companies themselves, but by government-funded institutions such as universities and the military.[28]

With regard specifically to HIV medications, the pharmaceutical companies and their trade association, the Pharmaceutical Researchers and Manufacturers of America (PhRMA), began to raise other claims that sometimes had a kernel of truth but seemed largely to be intended to obfuscate the question of pricing. The developing world lacked the infrastructural capacity to distribute drugs, they argued, even though there manifestly were many hospitals and pharmacies with empty shelves that could begin distributing medications immediately. The pharmaceutical companies also opined that medications produced in the developing world would be of unreliable quality and might even be shipped back to the developed world and unknowingly used there, even though generics from developing countries are manufactured, packaged and distributed in identifiably different ways. Perhaps most egregiously, it was suggested with little or no evidence that Africans lacked the ability to adhere to complex medication regimens, either for cultural reasons or because of their difficult life circumstances. Since poor medication adherence can promote drug resistance, it was argued that the continent might become a reservoir of drug-resistant HIV that would eventually spread to the developed world as well.

The pharmaceutical companies were adept at using their wealth, political influence, and their lawyers to threaten developing countries on multiple fronts. Given the magnitude of the AIDS epidemic in the developing world, however, it was perhaps inevitable that governments in the developing world would view the epidemic as a legitimate "national emergency" or "circumstance of extreme urgency" as outlined in Article 30 of TRIPS. Thailand and Brazil were among the first to begin publicly testing the waters, prompting the backlash from the pharmaceutical industry and threats of trade sanctions from the U.S. government that would lead to the first actions of a global movement to promote universal access to medications for people with HIV.

BRIDGING THE GAP?

Although the prevailing mood at the 1996 International AIDS Conference in Vancouver had been one of guarded optimism, the mood in many quarters two years later in Geneva was buoyant. The news of the preceding twenty-four months had revolutionized the epidemic, at least among those who could afford access to the new drugs—which it soon became clear would be fewer than 5 percent of the global population of those living with HIV. For the remaining 95 percent of those living with HIV, especially the more than thirty million in sub-Saharan Africa, the availability of HAART seemed to be almost a cruel joke.

Prior to 1996, both the developed and developing worlds had been united in their inability to stop HIV at either the societal or individual level, although the wealthier countries always had much greater abilities to prevent and treat opportunistic infections. A general mood of international cooperation and even commiseration had thus prevailed, with collaborations in such areas as vaccine research and prevention outreach that offered benefits to both sides. Still, in the absence of treatment options and in the face of intractable domestic problems, "international" AIDS activism consisted largely of interactions among activists based in developed nations and focused largely on their own domestic AIDS crises. Indeed, before 1996, globally oriented AIDS activism was limited mainly to a few vocal but small groups and individuals such as Paul Boneberg, leader of the Global AIDS Action Network (GAAN), and Eric Sawyer, founder of the Global AIDS Action Committee of ACT UP.

After 1996, however, a few forward-looking thinkers began to recognize the potential for a dramatic division of the world's population of people with AIDS between rich and poor camps. Perhaps the most prescient speech had been made at the Vancouver conference in 1996 by Harvard public health professor Jonathan Mann. As head of the World Health Organization's Special Program on AIDS, Mann had pioneered the application of human rights frameworks to the burgeoning global AIDS epidemic. Now, noting the erosion of the international solidarity that existed when both rich and poor nations were equally helpless before AIDS, Mann said:

In moving forward, we must challenge—boldly and without compromise—two of the most persuasive and powerful of all status quos. First, we must challenge the idea, which all too often passes for wisdom, that what is, is what must inevitably be. For we who are engaged against AIDS share a belief, indeed to be working against AIDS we must believe, that the world can change, that the future is not the inevitable consequence of the past, that the chains of pain and suffering we have inherited can be broken, that we can each contribute meaningfully to the healing of the world. We will also challenge a second fundamental status quo, the idea that we are each alone, independent, isolated beings.

We have the precious, historic opportunity here, now, today in Vancouver to start or accelerate a profound transformation in the movement against AIDS.... For the future of the global effort against AIDS is, as it has always been, literally in our hands. To create and build a new solidarity in the face of all the standard, historical, expected, routine and powerful status quos which seek to divide us; to contribute to that society transformation which offers hope against AIDS and for the world: this is a task—no, a destiny—worthy of our past, our aspirations, our commitment, our dignity, and our lives.[29]

By 1998, the gap between richer and poorer could no longer be overlooked or downplayed. "Two years have passed since the last international conference in Vancouver. These have been two years of progress, but these have also been two years in which we have seen the AIDS gap widen," said UNAIDS executive director Peter Piot at the 1998 Geneva conference. "The theme of our conference is 'Bridging the Gap.' The biggest AIDS gap of all is the gap between what we can do today, and what we are actually doing. It is my hope that this twelfth World Conference will mark the time when the global community commits itself to closing this AIDS gap. Now is the time for us to embrace a new realism and a new urgency in our efforts."[30]

Nonetheless, the mood after the Geneva conference was more one of frustration than of clear direction; the stirrings of cognitive liberation had not yet sparked a coherent movement. Jonathan Mann might have continued to provide the leadership for such a movement, but he and his wife were among the passengers aboard SwissAir Flight 111 which crashed off the coast of Nova Scotia in September 1998, killing all those aboard and depriving the movement of a major leader. Still, the evidence of a growing gap between the developed and developing worlds presented in Geneva had a profound impact on many others in attendance. Among them was New York AIDS physician Alan Berkman, who had a long and complicated history of social activism and organized resistance to injustice.

By 1998 Berkman was the medical director at Highbridge-Woodycrest, a residential care facility for people with AIDS in the Bronx, and a fellow at the Columbia University School of Public Health. But throughout the 1970s, Berkman had been at the forefront of New Left activism, publicly supporting militant groups such as the Weather Underground. Berkman's life took a dramatic turn when he treated the gunshot wounds that a member of the Weather Underground sustained in a shoot-out with police after robbing an armored car in Nyack, New York. When he did not turn her in to the police, Berkman became the first doctor charged for such actions since Dr. Samuel Mudd, who had treated the wounds of the fleeing John Wilkes Booth. Berkman refused to testify in the matter and was jailed for a year, after which he was indicted as an accessory after the fact to the armored car robbery, in which two policemen and a Brinks guard were killed. Berkman jumped bail and fled underground. After two years as a fugitive, Berkman was arrested in 1985 and spent the period from 1985 to 1992 in maximum-security prisons, including four years in solitary confinement. During that period he could only read about the expansion of the AIDS epidemic from his prison cell, but underwent two bouts of life-threatening Hodgkin's Disease which led him to a highly publicized battle for adequate medical treatment.[31]

In many ways, Berkman's work in AIDS drew upon his own experiences, both the firsthand dehumanizing experience of being incarcerated and denied adequate treatment as well as the ideological commitments which had led him first into medicine and later into radical politics. Six years after his release from prison and his start of hands-on work in combating HIV in New York City, Berkman visited South Africa as part of his work as a fellow at the Columbia School of Public Health. "In South Africa, I began to see the outlines of what was happening and what was going to happen around AIDS in Africa. Besides what we were looking at in the patients, I could tell from my clinical work that a fair percentage of the staff had AIDS," said Berkman.[32]

Then I went to the Geneva conference and experienced the inertia manifested by people who were supposed to be providing leadership around global AIDS. I saw people from the West walk out of the sessions that were about global AIDS. I was watching what Jonathan Mann had said might happen in front of my very eyes, sort of crystallized through the international AIDS conference. I saw the way that it always happens about the scientists and the doctors and some of the advocates from the U.S. being wined and dined and a lot of money being spent on marketing by the drug companies. By '98 they were triumphant—the cocktails were selling like hotcakes, as it were. And there seemed something almost so pornographic about it, having just come from Africa.[33]

Still in Geneva, Berkman began formulating an idea which "emerged from a sequence of events that took place over a finite period of time, obviously from the background of my life but also from the challenge that Jonathan Mann put out in Vancouver—are we going to let this split the solidarity that had existed?" The crystallizing experience of Berkman's vision, he acknowledges, would not seem out of place in a film or novel. "I visited Dachau, the concentration camp, and had these long train rides in Germany and then from Germany to Paris in which to sort of mull it over. And what the trip to Germany did was to say: we all ask why didn't someone do something at the time, and I kept saying there has to be something we can do."[34]

"And I really had this feeling that people were frustrated, people wanted to do something, happy to do something, but nobody gave people anything concrete to do. So it was all those trends together and it consolidated around the idea that we don't have to accept that treatment is impossible, because of the price at least," said Berkman. "The price is a man-made obstacle that we can change, and in the process of changing the price, I didn't know what else would change, but I really had a sense that that was something that we could do."[35] By that time, there was already hard evidence to back up Berkman's suspicion that pharmaceutical prices were wildly inflated. This evidence came from Brazil, where the government decided in 1997 to have its national pharmaceutical industry produce generic HIV drugs and these generic versions that were created cost less than a quarter of what was being charged by the pharmaceutical giants.[36]

Berkman was not alone in seeking to add a sense of urgency to "bridging the gap." By the time of the Vancouver conference, John James had been publishing his highly influential newsletter *AIDS Treatment News* since 1988, at a time when AIDS treatments had still seemed a distant prospect. Many of the same forward-looking qualities that caused him to embrace the cause of AIDS treatment in the mid-1980s had by the mid-1990s enabled him to imagine an activist response to the cause of global AIDS treatment access. "Imagine the effect on trade policy regarding pharmaceutical patents if Congress and the president repeatedly got thousands of letters from constituents—and major religious, medical, political, and other leaders around the world spoke out," wrote James in a widely circulated e-mail in September 1998. "Would the companies even push for policies that killed people if, when they did, the human consequences and the specific companies and officials involved were prominently reported?"[37]

Writing two months later in *AIDS Treatment News,* James formalized his reasoning. "Even without changing the GATT treaty itself, it would be surprisingly feasible for an activist movement to save lives. . . . Congress, the White House, the U.S. Trade Representative, and others usually hear from only one side—multinational corporations, their industry associations, and organizations which have been created, paid, or pressured to echo their line. Usually *no one* addresses any other side—effectively turning the U.S. government into a tool of corporate interests," wrote James. Although a mass movement would be best, "even a far smaller movement could restrain some of the worst excesses, by exposing abuses and forcing debate on the merits. If Federal agencies heard not only from industry, but from churches, doctors and other medical professionals, activists, and others— and from the press as well—much would be different."[38]

James formulated these ideas in part through his contacts with economist Jamie Love, director of the Consumer Project on Technology (CPTech), a Washington DC–based organization founded by consumer advocate Ralph Nader that was active in areas as diverse as electronic commerce, telecommunications, and antitrust enforcement and policy. One of Love's areas of specialization was health care and intellectual property rights, particularly the TRIPS framework. By 1998, Love, his associate Rob Weissman at the affiliated organization Essential Action, and others at CPTech were involved with assisting the South African government in its attempts to access affordable medications, attempts which were being thwarted by the U.S. government.[39]

In an interview with James, Love made clear that from his professional vantage point, AIDS activists had a strong basis under international law upon which to make their demands. "The problem for developing countries is not whether compulsory licensing of pharmaceuticals is legal, because it clearly is legal. It's the political problem of whether they will face sanctions from the United States government, for doing things they have a legal right to do but which the United States government does not like." Love noted that in South Africa, the United States was "trying to stop the South African government from doing compulsory licensing of essential medicines for South Africa, not because it's against international law, but because U.S. pharmaceutical companies, and English, German, and Swiss pharmaceutical companies don't like it." Love added that U.S. trade policy was not even in accord with principles enshrined in American law. Instead, he argued, the United States used as its standard "the wish list of policies that are dreamed up by the International Federation of Pharmaceutical Manufacturers Associations."[40]

A CALL TO ACTION

The concerns raised by Berkman, thus, were also being articulated by John James, Jamie Love, and a growing body of public health practitioners, activists, consumer advocates, and others. But it was Berkman who first formalized his thoughts into a call to action. "Many felt that the gap grew wider at Geneva. One possible explanation for the sense of frustration and futility that many felt was that 14,000 concerned individuals gathered at a cost of millions of dollars, were confronted by the global realities, and left with no clear sense of goals, priorities or strategies," wrote Berkman a few months later, drawing explicitly on the speech delivered by Jonathan Mann in Vancouver in 1996. Berkman then led the way in issuing a call "to initiate a multi-level strategy rooted in grassroots activism, to demand that the private sector, in cooperation with governments and non-governmental agencies, take concrete steps to dramatically expand access to life-sustaining medications, nutrients and nutritional supplements to HIV-infected individuals around the world." Eschewing the "profit-loss statement" approach of the pharmaceutical companies, Berkman continued, "The rationale for demanding greater access to antiretroviral agents and those medications that treat tuberculosis and opportunistic infections is clear: they extend life. ... Even if only parts of this program were adopted, the survival benefits would be dramatic."[41]

Setting out what would become the basic outlines of the global AIDS treatment activist agenda, he called for immediate "drastic bulk discount or outright donations" of medications, followed by establishing "a price that would remove cost as a defining factor in a country's ability to treat their population." Over the longer term, Berkman called for companies to "relinquish [patent rights] on a negotiated basis to countries that have the capacity to produce pharmaceuticals and which fall below certain per capital income levels." And, finally, addressing concerns about pharmaceutical company profits, Berkman noted: "the current reality is that the vast majority of profits on pharmaceuticals come from the countries of the North. Voluntarily allowing regional production of these products would result in little direct loss for drug companies."[42]

This last point was a particular source of outrage for Berkman and other activists: the pharmaceutical companies were not even defending actual profits but rather simply their patent rights in the abstract. Indeed, Berkman and others came to suspect that the pharmaceutical companies' true agenda was closely guarding their actual cost of manufacture. Their fear, it was becoming increasingly clear, was that production of low-cost generic medications would decisively reveal the enormous mark-ups built into their prices—perhaps provoking "blowback" in the form of increasing demands for lower drug prices in the developed world.[43]

Although the issue of drug prices was center stage in the nascent treatment access movement, the activists were well aware that the global AIDS crisis is a multidimensional problem, involving questions of prevention, vaccine development, sex education, women's rights, poverty reduction, and a host of other issues. But a consensus was reached early on that treatment was not only the most urgent imperative, but also the one that would be the most likely to garner wider support. "I think we correctly grasped the fact that the availability of treatment humanized the issue of global AIDS in a particular way," said Berkman. "It was more concrete in that you could actually save lives and in that way more compelling. If we talked about everything we really need to deal with the global AIDS epidemic, we would lose focus and not accomplish anything. And focusing on treatment had a passion to it that was different than prevention. If there was going to be a change in global AIDS policy, we needed to mobilize a base, and in the affected countries, treatment speaks differently to people, it's very clear that it's about saving lives, about saying that you couldn't just write off 35 million people."[44]

Berkman's impassioned call to action around the question of drug pricing was widely circulated within preexisting public health and activist networks, particularly in New York and along the East Coast, leading to a series of biweekly conference calls beginning in January 1999. The new working group brought together an eclectic group of AIDS activists, public health practitioners, consumer rights, human rights, and free-trade advocates along with individuals such as doctors, economists, academics, and journalists. Adopting the image of "bridging the gap," the new organization assumed the name the Health Global Access Project Coalition, later simply "Health GAP."[45]

Among the founding individuals and organizations of the coalition were Jamie Love of CPTech and John James of *AIDS Treatment News*. A number of other people and groups with long histories in the AIDS and gay and lesbian rights arenas, as well as public health and human rights more broadly, were also early members of the Health GAP Coalition. Among these earliest participants were[46]

- The International Gay and Lesbian Human Rights Commission (IGLHRC), a New York–based nongovernmental association that uses human rights instruments and international grassroots advocacy to oppose discrimination or abuse on the basis of sexual orientation or expression, gender identity or expression, and/or HIV status. IGLHRC staff members Sidney Levy and Karyn Kaplan were early Health GAP members.
- Mobilization Against AIDS (MAA), a San Francisco–based AIDS advocacy and educational organization. A key early player in Health GAP was MAA's director Donna Rae Palmer.
- The AIDS Treatment Data Network, a community-based organization in New York offering treatment access and advocacy, case management, supportive counseling, and information services to HIV-positive people with limited resources.
- Essential Action, an organization promoting citizen participation and affiliated with CPTech in Washington DC and codirected by Robert Weissman.
- Search for a Cure, a Boston-based group dedicated to promoting education and advocacy for safe and effective HIV treatments.

A number of other large preexisting nongovernmental organizations served as close collaborators without formally becoming members of the Health GAP Coalition. Among these were Médecins san Frontières, the French-founded international humanitarian aid organization providing emergency medical assistance; Health Action International, a global network seeking to increase access and improve the rational use of essential medicines; Partners in Health, a health advocacy organization working predominantly in the Caribbean; the Treatment Action Campaign, an AIDS activist organization based in South Africa; and ACT UP Paris, which was unique among ACT UP chapters in adopting a structure that included paid staff.[47]

If much of the professional expertise and institutional connections were offered by these various nongovernmental organizations and their staff, much of the tactical expertise and organizational capability came from individuals who were mobilized through the old ACT UP network in the United States. Although ACT UP was largely moribund, the institutional and interpersonal linkages from the domestic activist heyday years earlier enabled news of the global initiatives to race through the activist community.

Broadly speaking, ACT UP had begun a precipitous decline after 1992, and many of its chapters had disbanded. To some activists, the advent of antiretroviral medications in 1996 had made the group seem all the more obsolete. By March of 1997, on the occasion of the tenth anniversary of ACT UP's founding, the *New York Times* wrote "the organization is a shadow of its former self. That devolution reflects the deaths of many of its leaders, the infighting that fractured the group, the seemingly inevitable mellowing of any radical movement, and the degree to which the armies that amassed to battle AIDS traveled a spectrum of grief from anger to acceptance. But more interesting, it demonstrates the extent to which protestors once clamoring at the dining room door have gained a place at the table."[48]

Yet even as many chapters had closed up shop and handed their files over to library collections, others managed to stay alive and even to reinvent themselves. Perhaps the most striking case was the near-death and then dramatic rebirth of ACT UP Philadelphia. By 1996, "the group was almost extinct. As was the case with other chapters, the gay men who'd founded ACT UP Philadelphia had either died or were so pleased with the new drugs that they no longer saw the need for political activism." The group had dwindled to just twelve active participants, but a core of four members—Kate Krauss, Asia Russell, Julie Davids, and Paul Davis—took a different tack, reorienting toward the needs of the often underserved people of color and injecting drug users who were rapidly becoming the "new face of AIDS."

The emerging new core of ACT UP Philadelphia found members of the city's large black community to be particularly receptive to their message about fighting AIDS in Africa, both because of feelings of ethnic solidarity as well as bonds of personal experience. "One reason the global AIDS struggle has resonated so deeply with our members is because of the shared experience. Our members know what it means to have shoddy health care. Our members know what it means not to be able to afford lifesaving drugs," explained Davis.[49] By forming alliances within the city's large urban minority population, the chapter was able to recapture the kind of support not seen for years, including protest events drawing up to 1,500 participants on a fleet of chartered buses. In a stark shift from the earlier largely white gay male profile of ACT UP, most of these protest participants were low-income African American heterosexuals.[50]

This same ethos directed ACT UP Philadelphia beyond the borders of the United States to turn their attention to sub-Saharan Africa. Their awareness of the AIDS crisis in Africa grew after they began receiving e-mails from activists in Zimbabwe who reported that morgues were being kept open twenty-four hours a day due to the huge influx of corpses, and that teenage girls were being infected by HIV-positive men who believed that they could be cured by having intercourse with virgins.[51] "To remain relevant, we've really had to follow the AIDS epidemic. It's not accurate to say we've gone somewhere else because things are all fixed here. But the corporate denial of medication to 25 million Africans reso- nates deeply with our members who have fought the same battles here," said Paul Davis.[52]

In New York, the onetime flagship chapter of ACT UP had continued to hold weekly meetings throughout the 1990s, but had dwindled greatly. Individual activists remained deeply involved with AIDS as an issue, how- ever, and remained able to tap into the accumulated experience. A key early player in Health GAP was Eric Sawyer, a founder of ACT UP New York and by the late 1990s the director of the HIV/AIDS and Human Rights Project. HIV-positive since 1981, Sawyer had long been on the cutting edge of both the United States and international AIDS activism, founding the Global AIDS Action Committee of ACT UP in 1991 and calling for multitiered pricing policies as early as the Vancouver conference. For Sawyer and some other members of ACT UP, the domestic and global epidemics were inseparable: "I am an international treatment activist today because I am angry that my friends in the developing world are dying due to lack of access to the treatments and health care I rely on to thrive with a fatal disease," Sawyer wrote in 2002. "I am an international treatment activist because I was born with a sense of humanity that tells me that every life matters and deserves to be fought for."[53]

Other ACT UP New York members who participated in early Health GAP actions included Mel Stewart, Mark Milano, Staci Smith, Bob Lederer, and Sharonann Lynch. Their influence would soon steer Health GAP onto the passionate and often confrontational path earlier blazoned by ACT UP. As Lynch explained, "Health GAP was an offshoot of earlier AIDS activism, especially when you look at its tactics. It borrowed the 'name and shame' tactic of ACT UP, it borrowed the strategy that if you are trying to bring about the end of the AIDS crisis, you do so by knocking down one barrier at a time. And you do that with the under-standing that not only are people dying, but that people are dying need-lessly. And why are there needless deaths? Because there's bad policy. And who's behind the bad policy? Bad policymakers. That's the premise, the working style of both ACT UP and Health GAP."[54]

TAKING ACTION

Thus, by 1999 key segments of the AIDS treatment activism community in the United States had begun to become both critically aware and crucially concerned about those living with HIV in the developing world who were being denied access to the antiretroviral medications. In April of that year, the Health GAP Coalition undertook its first formal activity, joining 1,500 protesters against the free trade-oriented Africa Growth and Opportunity Act (AGOA). Health GAP members took the lead to coordinate media coverage of AGOA's negative impact and supported instead an African trade bill proposed by Rep. Jesse Jackson, Jr.[55] Shortly thereafter, eight activists disrupted the AGOA vote on the floor of the House of Representatives, stalling the chamber for ten minutes by chaining themselves to a balcony and chanting while unfurling a banner reading "AFRICA IS NOT FOR SALE."[56]

With their inaugural activity behind them, Health GAP sought out opportunities to apply political pressure through bold direct action, but at first the prospects seemed to be few. Both houses of Congress were controlled by Republicans whose principal preoccupation was cutting taxes and curbing deficit spending. Few of these Republican leaders were susceptible to pressure from AIDS activists, and many had long been hostile to both foreign aid and funding for AIDS causes. Democratic senators and representatives, particularly those with large African American and gay constituencies, were more responsive but had comparatively little leverage; being in the minority in both the Senate and the House of Repre-sentatives, they chaired not a single Congressional committee and could only affect legislation at the margins.

Prospects for influence on the Clinton administration might have seemed better, but Clinton himself was preoccupied by the protracted Monica Lewinsky scandal and his eventual impeachment; in the period 1998–1999, he was at the nadir of his power and influence. In any case, not only was he moving to the political center for years but he was also ineli-gible for reelection and hence unusually shielded from public pressure. Then AIDS activists hit upon their first great domestic political opportu-nity: the presidential campaign of Al Gore.

At the time, Gore was seeking to shore up his support among core Democratic constituencies against a primary challenge from the left of former Senator Bill Bradley, as well as a vague threat from even further to the left from Ralph Nader running with the Green Party. Not only was Gore thus the most vulnerable senior member of the Clinton administration, but he also, coincidentally, had headed a binational commission with South African deputy president (and later president) Thabo Mbeki in which many of the substantive issues of bilateral U.S.–South African relations were discussed. It was through this commission that Gore had in 1997 and 1998 threatened South Africa with U.S. trade sanctions if it were to violate the strict U.S. interpretation of international patent law. At the time, South Africa was planning to issue a compulsory license that would allow its domestic pharmaceutical industry to produce low-cost generic versions of brand-name antiretroviral medications.[57] Gore was already being singled out by the South African protest group Treatment Action Campaign (TAC),[58] but his role as the Clinton administration's enforcer had gone largely unnoticed in the United States.

So why did the Clinton administration more broadly seek to impose such a highly restrictive definition of international patent rights, a definition that disregarded the established right of countries facing a public health emergency to break patents? As one commentator noted, "The motivation here is easy to decipher. Patents on pharmaceutical drugs bring in some $75–80 billion a year to U.S. drug manufacturers. These patents create a legal monopoly for the companies that own them, and they will go to great lengths to protect their monopolies and extend them to the farthest corners of the earth. One of the things they do is contribute a small percentage of their monopoly profits to U.S. political candidates and parties, thereby enlisting the federal government in their cause."[59]

With the TRIPS framework new and largely untested, the governments of Thailand and South Africa sought to exercise their Article 30 rights. Thailand wished to issue a compulsory license for the manufacture of the antiretroviral drug didanosine (ddI). South Africa went further by passing the sweeping South African Medicines and Medical Regulatory Devices Act designed to combat the multiple health problems besetting the post-apartheid population through both compulsory licensing and parallel importing. The response was swift—the office of the U.S. Trade Representative threatened both nations with trade sanctions, that is to say high tariffs that would cut off their ability to competitively export products into the U.S. market. Thailand backed down, but South Africa held its ground and found itself on "a watchlist" and with its benefits under the Generalized System of Preferences suspended.[60] The stage was set for a major confrontation, with critics charging that the United States government was not only enforcing the TRIPS, but taking extra steps they dubbed "TRIPS plus."

Hence for both tactical and substantive reasons, Gore became the focus of attention from the Health GAP Coalition. According to founder Alan Berkman: "We didn't target Gore out of any particular desire to influence the election. What we wanted to influence, and did, was U.S. trade policy. I think we correctly decided that Gore was the right person to focus on."[61] It was in mid-June 1999 that the policy expertise and the finely honed protest skills gathered together in Health GAP were first merged to launch a full-scale demand for attention on the Gore campaign.

"GORE'S GREED KILLS!"

The targeting of the Gore campaign began with a hastily called meeting of about twenty New York–based activists, including several leaders of the emerging Health GAP Coalition. Mark Milano, a longtime ACT UP member, became a key player in the Gore zaps despite having limited his activism largely to U.S. domestic issues throughout the 1990s. "I personally didn't get involved with global treatment activism before '99—and I think that a lot of people in the U.S. didn't—because it seemed sort of impossible," said Milano. "But I was furious about this situation. This was different—this was an African government taking steps itself to provide HIV treatment in a very concrete way that would have a tremendous impact on the health of its people. And my government was preventing them from doing that. It was a situation ripe for action—I wasn't some outsider telling South Africa what to do. They had taken the lead, and I could tell my government: 'Back off—you are not the cop of the world.' I felt I could do something as an American that would help people around the world."[62]

Drawing on a decade's worth of experience in political protest, the activists knew instinctively that Gore would be at his most vulnerable during the speech in his hometown of Carthage, Tennessee, at which he would officially announce his candidacy for the presidency. The event would be saturated in media coverage, full of cameras eager to find a spark of the unexpected in the otherwise tightly scripted event. And so a handful of activists decided to travel to Carthage, most making the sixteen-hour road trip from New York, and then found a way to slip into the campaign launch event and work their way to the front of the room.[63]

Although the Gore zaps were officially carried out under the ad hoc name "AIDS Drugs for Africa" and in coordination with Health GAP,

the protests were vintage ACT UP. A joint press release from the New
York and Philadelphia chapters of ACT UP described the unfolding events:

Shouting "Gore kills Africans," blowing whistles and waving signs and banners
demanding "AIDS drugs for Africa," about a dozen AIDS activists stunned United
States Vice President Al Gore at each of his first three stops to kick off his presidential campaign. . . . Seven activists interrupted Gore's Carthage, Tennessee
speech with whistles and yelling, causing Gore to stop in mid-thought, remain
silent and open-mouthed for a few seconds, before gathering his wits enough to
proclaim his support of free speech. . . . [In Manchester, New Hampshire], another
half dozen activists found seats on the stage just a few feet away from Gore. As he
started to speak, they stood, unfurled a banner demanding AIDS drugs for Africa
and chanted for about a minute. . . . Gore said repeatedly, as the activists stood next
to him and chanted, "I'll be happy to meet with you later." . . . Subsequently,
Clinton administration officials and friends have called the activists and their colleagues sounding desperate to find out how they can stop the demonstrations,
which have clearly embarrassed Gore. Activists are repeating their demands for
a reversal of administration policy on access to affordable drugs.[64]

Media attention was considerable, particularly since it was hardly "news"
that Gore was running for president, and since his campaigning style was so
lackluster. "If Al Gore had been a better campaigner, would we have gotten as
much attention?," asked Berkman. "I don't know, but we were the most
interesting things happening on his campaign for a while. . . . So what happened was that the Bradley people wanted to talk to us, the Republican head of
one of the subcommittees that then looked into U.S. foreign policy on AIDS
asked if we would testify about it. The Presidential Advisory Commission on
AIDS felt they had to ask us. . . . We met with the Gore campaign also."[65]

In true ACT UP style, pressure remained unrelenting. The activists had
soon dubbed Gore's election bid the "Apartheid 2000 Campaign" and mobilized en masse on June 28 at a Gore fundraising dinner in Philadelphia. Featuring a life-sized Gore marionette whose strings were held by pharmaceutical
company executives, the protestors demanded that "Gore must cease threats
of trade sanctions against South Africa and other developing nations that are
attempting to provide access to essential AIDS medications" as well as other
steps toward increasing drug access.[66] The protests also helped to prompt a
letter from the Congressional Black Caucus to Gore, to which Gore replied,
"I support South Africa's effort to provide AIDS drugs at reduced prices
through compulsory licensing and parallel importing, so long as they are
carried out in a way that is consistent with international agreements."[67]

The activists were at first skeptical; Asia Russell of ACT UP Philadelphia
said of Gore's letter, "This statement is smoke and mirrors. Al Gore could

do so much more than this statement. He could do a lot to clarify the position of the administration in terms of reversing policies that are in action now."[68] But to the surprise of many, the Clinton administration did indeed go on to do just that, lifting the threat of trade sanctions against South Africa less than ninety days after the protests began and undertaking a number of other concessions.[69]

Still, the activists kept up their pressure, shifting their focus from the Gore campaign to the office of U.S. Trade Representative (USTR) Charlene Barshefsky. On October 6, ACT UP organized a 750-person demonstration at the USTR office in Washington DC. Even more dramatically, on the morning of November 17, days before a scheduled ministerial meeting of the World Trade Organization in Seattle, "AIDS activists from ACT UP and other groups stormed and occupied her office on the second floor of the USTR building. Another five climbers chained themselves to her balcony with a large banner demanding 'Essential Medication for all Nations.' The demonstrators threw dollar bills featuring Barshefsky's image, and empty pill bottles symbolizing the effect of USTR bullying of nations hard-hit by HIV/AIDS."[70] Barshefsky later revealed that she had been surprised by the issues raised by the activists: "I was certainly not aware of this at all. . . . In years past, this issue was treated purely as a trade issue and an intellectual property rights issue."[71]

Mere days after the second USTR action, Clinton announced that it was official U.S. policy to no longer threaten trade sanctions against any African country that pursued compulsory licensing or parallel importing; this statement was written into a formal Executive Order the following May.[72] Going further still, however, Gore was also given the task of announcing "the largest-ever increase in the U.S. commitment to international AIDS programs—$100 million to fight AIDS in Africa, India and other areas."[73] The Clinton administration also designated AIDS as a threat to national security, thus creating an entirely new line of argumentation for addressing the global epidemic. Continuing this focus, in January 2000, Gore addressed a UN Security Council session on AIDS in Africa (this was the first time a U.S. vice president did so and the first such session to focus on a health issue). "We must do much more to provide basic care and treatment to the growing number of people who, thank God, are living, instead of dying, with HIV and AIDS. Today, fewer than five percent of those living with AIDS in Africa have access to even basic care," said Gore at the UN before announcing another $100 million in global AIDS funding and an additional $50 million for vaccine development.[74]

In all, the rapid reversal of the trade policies of the Clinton administration in the aftermath of the Gore and USTR zaps provided stunning evidence that focused AIDS treatment activism could alter an entrenched status quo. Within the span of a few months, the U.S. government went from being a principal obstacle to access to AIDS drugs in the developing world to one of its major proponents. These quick policy victories appear to have had much the same catalytic effect for Health GAP and global treatment access movement that the Montgomery bus boycott had on the civil rights movement—transforming a nascent idea into a burgeoning movement by demonstrating that a relative handful of committed activists really could effect change on a literally global scale.

In his book about global AIDS, *The Invisible People,* author Greg Behrman presents evidence that by the time of the Gore zaps, the Clinton administration in general, and Gore's office in particular, had already begun secretly working on ways to ease pressure on South Africa and other developing countries with regard to pharmaceutical patents.[75] This preexisting groundwork may help to explain why the reaction of the administration was coordinated so quickly; the pace of policy change is rarely so abrupt. But the crucial catalytic role of activist pressure also seems irrefutable, and it is impossible to say how, when, or even whether the Clinton administration would actually have changed their positions on the issue of pharmaceutical patents without pressure from activists. Gore himself begrudgingly conceded their role. "This tragedy has outstripped all of the efforts to stop it, and that's why we're now asking the rest of the world community to join us as we redouble out efforts," he said at the time of UN Security Council meeting. "The (AIDS) activists were right that this was ignored for far too long."[76]

THE BATTLE OF SEATTLE AND BEYOND

Not entirely coincidentally, the 1999 activist demonstrations against the Gore campaign coincided with the launching of a widescale anti-globalization movement in the United States and abroad which would serve as the next vehicle for protest action around AIDS in the developing world. Indeed it was at the start of the WTO meeting in Seattle that Clinton announced the formal change in U.S. trade policy regarding AIDS medications. Of course, that meeting would later go on to become better known as the site of massive street protests that first brought the anti-globalization movement to wide-scale public attention. Although not all agree, some already consider the so-called Battle of Seattle a major watershed event: "November 30, 1999 marked a turning point in history. Tens of thousands of ordinary citizens took to the streets of Seattle to stop the World Trade Organization from conducting 'business as usual.' . . . We can now envision the formation of a truly global movement capable of challenging the most powerful institutions on the planet."[77]

Much like Health GAP, the Seattle antiglobalization protestors represented a broad activist coalition: "Contrary to the negative portrayal in the corporate media, the protestors were organized, educated, and determined. They were human rights activists, labor activists, indigenous people, people of faith, steel workers and farmers. They were forest activists, environmentalists, social justice workers, students and teachers."[78] People concerned with global AIDS have been prominent within the ranks of the protestors at Seattle and subsequently in such sites as Washington DC, Prague, Genoa, and even Doha in Qatar. Beyond finding new common ground, some have claimed that the antiglobalization movement is in some ways rooted in earlier AIDS activism; an anthology published in 2002 was even entitled *From ACT UP to the WTO*.[79]

By 1999 "fighting the AIDS pandemic had come to mean fighting institutionalized racism, sexism, and the class system, in addition to homophobia [and] fighting undemocratic international trade laws, an unjust immigration system, the prison industrial complex, poverty, unresponsive government, budget cuts, a disaster in health care, and countless other manifestations of bureaucracies that put profits ahead of people," wrote AIDS activist Ben Shepherd. "Oppressions overlap and influence each other as do movements. This insight is the essential kernel of the story of activism from ACT UP to the WTO."[80]

The impact of the Seattle protests was twofold. First, they brought the dark side of globalization front and center into the consciousness of the global public. Until then, globalization remained a vague notion seemingly disconnected from the lives of ordinary people. Although debate over the NAFTA treaty in the early 1990s had raised some concerns about possible loss of jobs in the United States, issues of globalization were generally portrayed as benign yet inevitable extensions of the triumph of democratic capitalism in the post–Cold War era. For the first time in full public view, the raucous protests of Seattle advanced the thesis that "free" trade was not necessarily "fair" trade, that capitalism could not be counted upon to protect natural resources, that corporate revenues would not always "trickle down" to those below, and that the social and economic rights of workers are often viewed as mere hindrances to profit maximization. Although the war was by no means won, the battle had been joined—and public opinion in the developed world became more attuned and receptive to the criticisms and critiques of globalization offered by antiwar, environmental, labor, human rights—and AIDS—activists.

Second, the Seattle protests dramatically accelerated the formation of networks of like-minded activists that were global in scope and focused on global issues. The heterogeneity of the protestors alone suggested the breadth of the antiglobalization movement and underscored the linkages among different issues areas. And shortly after Seattle, a global alliance began to take shape drawing together AIDS activists not only from North America and Western Europe but also Brazil, Thailand, South Africa, and other countries and regions of the globe. This merging of the U.S.-based AIDS treatment activist movement into a larger transnational issue advocacy network is the principal subject of Part II of this book.

Part II

Forging a Global AIDS Treatment Activist Network

Introduction

The U.S.-based treatment access movement that took off with the Gore protests and found common cause with the antiglobalization activists flooding the streets of Seattle moved rapidly in the first two years of the new millennium. This period was marked with a stream of victories that cumulatively reversed the ideological position of governments and individuals around the world. Global treatment access went from being conceived as an impractical, utopian wish to a moral imperative. And yet, events also reflected the wisdom in the old adage "be careful what you wish for." By January 2003 even the president of the United States was promoting AIDS plans, including treatment components, on a scale previously unimaginable within the Washington development community. Having won the initial engagement—in terms of broadly changing the terms of how the global AIDS pandemic should be addressed—the movement, and key organizations within it like Health GAP, have had to face a surprising number of remaining battles. Some of these battles were the inevitable consequence of victory. Like every movement, this one has had to reflect on what remains to be done in order to convert a major rhetorical victory into concrete changes on the ground. Other battles have reflected the changes that have occurred because of outside events, particularly the terrorist attacks of September 11, which destroyed many of the political opportunities of the movement by simultaneously elevating national security above other policy issues and making the protest-based tactics of the movement more difficult, politically and practically.

Part II of this book takes a closer look at this trajectory from victory to the more problematic quest of implementing and institutionalizing gains in an inhospitable political environment. Chapter 3 focuses on a relatively short period of time—from July 2000 to June 2001. During this chronologically brief but substantively critical period, the potential of the global

treatment access movement became readily apparent. A number of circumstances fell into place including the dramatic fall in the price of AIDS
medicines, because of aggressive generic marketing, the creation of a
new global drug purchasing mechanism, and two major international meetings on HIV/AIDS that facilitated contact among activists and their allies.
The period was also marked by heavy domestic activity within a number of
AIDS-affected countries including South Africa, Brazil, and Kenya, as activists targeted their own governments and/or private sector opponents. All
of this activity helped to form, and was in turn supported by, the formation
of a transnational advocacy network dedicated to the goal of addressing the
global AIDS crisis by ensuring the availability of treatment for all.

In their defining work on these networks Margaret Keck and Kathryn
Sikkink note that they are "characterized by voluntary, reciprocal and
horizontal patterns of communication and exchange" and that network
members "share values and frequently exchange information and services."[1] In the case of the global treatment access network these communication patterns and exchanges have been hugely facilitated by
globalization processes, particularly global communication systems including e-mail, cell phones, and fax machines, and global transportation systems
that have facilitated international conferences and meetings. It is not cir-
cumstantial that the rise of this transnational network coincided with the
time frame in which inaccessibility to AIDS medications was most vigorously challenged and publicly questioned, and that key players, from world
leaders to government bureaucrats and finally the pharmaceutical industry
itself, began to shift their positions. How this happened, and particularly
how the transnational advocacy network was able to connect, amplify, and
build upon victories, is the central narrative of Chapter 3.

Chapter 4 picks up the narrative in the aftermath of September 11,
2001—after terrorists had destroyed the World Trade Center and consequently set in motion a host of events and reactions that would have enormous consequences in many areas—including the global treatment access
movement. Contrary to fears at the time, September 11 did not signal the
death knell of the treatment activist movement, but it did add major complications to the tactics, strategies, and outcomes of treatment activism. In
fact, several of the most significant accomplishments of the movement
occurred post–September 11. As Chapter 4 will detail, a dramatic new global
AIDS program was unveiled by the U.S. government in early 2003, and
significant progress was made on some multilateral measures as well. Yet
other major initiatives and legislation undertaken after September 11—
including the USA PATRIOT Act, the Iraq War, and the overall financial

and political emphasis on internal and external security—have made pushing a global AIDS agenda (let alone a more specialized global treatment access agenda) much more difficult. Strategically, the competition against AIDS as an issue worthy of public and policymaker attention has grown exponentially, while tactically, organizational work within such a protest-based movement has become much more complicated. Legally, the PATRIOT Act and other antiterrorism measures have made protest and especially civil disobedience activities more risky and difficult. A more intangible but still real complication is the shift in the mood of the country, which has appreciably lowered public tolerance of criticism of the U.S. government and its policies, especially when it is made using confrontational tactics. The fourth chapter of the book examines the victories that occur in this contradictory landscape, and also looks at the fundamental dilemma created for the movement by these victories—namely, what should the movement do once it has won, at least rhetorically, its central goal?

TRANSNATIONAL ADVOCACY NETWORKS

The first part of the book explicitly draws inspiration from the McAdam political process model. This model continues to offer important theoretical insights for the movement once it moves from a domestic to a global focus. In his discussion of expanded political opportunities, McAdam notes that one of the ways they facilitate political opportunity is by "increasing the political leverage of a single insurgent group."[2] Either of these two developments will, in turn, help challenger groups in two ways: first by increasing their strength and in turn their bargaining position, and second, by raising the costs of repressing insurgent action.[3] The strengthening of the leverage of insurgents was occurring repeatedly because of both changes to the political opportunity structure (such as the lowering of drug prices by agents allied with, but not groups within, the activist movement) and victories that serve as foundations for expanded campaigns.

At this point a second and newer model, specifically developed around global activism, serves as a critical interpretive framework. This is the vision of the transnational advocacy network developed by Keck and Sikkink. In examining the interactions within world politics Keck and Sikkink see three types of transnational networks: networks of economic actors and firms, networks of scientists and experts bound by professional ties and shared views on the causality and solutions of policy problems (also known as epistemic communities), and activists whose network formation is motivated by shared values and principles.[4] It is this final group that comprises the transnational advocacy networks on which they focus, and which the global treatment activist movement clearly exemplifies.

In their discussion of the major actors that comprise transnational advocacy networks, they suggest seven potential categories, not all of which must be present. They include some predictable groups, such as domestic and international nongovernmental organizations (NGOs) dedicated to research and advocacy, as well as local social movements, churches, unions, consumer groups, and intellectuals. But they also may include foundations, the media, parts of regional and international intergovernmental organizations (IGOs), and perhaps most surprisingly, parts of the executive and/or parliamentary branches of government.[5] These networks, comprised of a variety of different actors but united by shared values and principles, use four main types of tactics. The first of these, *information politics*, relies on the capability of activists to generate timely, credible, and useful information and to disseminate it to wherever it will have most impact. This information, though it must be accurate, is not meant to be neutral; rather it can serve as an alternative source for the media, the public, and policymakers, and can be framed as narratives and as a different presentation of problems and solutions. Keck and Sikkink cite the example of anti–infant formula campaigners who used information about how corporate sales were leading to declines in breast feeding and consequent rises in infant malnutrition and mortality to paint Nestlé as "baby killers." *Symbolic politics* uses symbols and stories to interpret events for a sometimes-distant target audience. Potent individuals, events, and images can become representative of larger issues, and can simplify complicated phenomena. *Leverage politics* pushes powerful actors to act in situations where weaker members of the network cannot, and *accountability politics* attempt to hold powerful actors to previous commitments and policy statements. Leverage may be material, as when human rights groups are able to get policymakers to cut off aid to regimes that violate human rights, or it may be moral, relying on the "mobilization of shame," as when campaigners seek to embarrass states or international organizations for not living up to previous commitments or stated values.

All of these tactics have been used, often in combination, by the global treatment access movement. A hallmark of the ACT UP chapters which still operate in the United States and Europe, and which helped to spawn Health GAP, has been the deft use of information politics, in the form of both savvy, specific policy papers and highly visible, accessible public information in the form of leaflets, posters, and handouts. Importantly, both the domestic and international AIDS movements have also understood that a key to information dissemination is coverage in the mainstream press. Hence, civil disobedience, die-ins, and other high-profile direct actions are usually well advertised to media outlets in advance, and when reporters arrive they are given extensive press packets and access to activist spokespeople.

Similarly, symbolic politics have been powerful tools in the AIDS arsenal from the time it was a domestic movement, from the pink triangle in a black background that came to symbolize ACT UP, to the political funerals and die-ins that were frequently employed to symbolize the devastation and suffering caused by government inaction. When the treatment access movement went global, the symbolic arsenal of the activists got even larger. Zackie Achmat, chair of South Africa's Treatment Action Coalition (TAC), who went on a "treatment fast" to publicize the unavailability of free AIDS medicines from the public center, is himself a powerful symbol to AIDS advocates and the global public. So, too, is TAC, which successfully used David and Goliath imagery in portraying its battle in league with the South African government against the powerful and well-financed international pharmaceutical industry over South Africa's right to promote public health over intellectual property protection.

Both leverage and accountability politics have also been highly successfully employed, often in combination. This happened in the targeting of Gore, who was in a prime position to affect the Clinton administration's trade policies with both South Africa and other countries generally. Moral leverage particularly has been a major tactical tool of the global treatment activist network, as it has variously shamed the pharmaceutical industry and governments, particularly the U.S. government, for blocking access of developing countries to affordable medications, and a variety of donor sources—again with the U.S. government at the top of the list—for failing to provide adequate financial resources for coping with the pandemic. No government, corporation, or international agency wants to be shown to have blood on its hands, a charge that has been successfully leveled against all these entities in the drive to push them to respond with greater urgency.

FORMING AN AIDS TREATMENT TRANSNATIONAL ADVOCACY NETWORK

Keck and Sikkink note that transnational advocacy networks are most likely to form under three conditions. The first is when domestic actors are blocked from accessing and impacting their own governments and resort to the "boomerang" pattern of using external allies to pressure their governments from outside. In other words, when activists find their rights violated or ignored by their own governments, they may seek allies who are citizens of other states to pressure *their* governments (and in some cases, third party organizations) to put pressure on the government that is guilty of the rights abuses. A second possibility occurs when activists actively promote networks because they believe it will promote their goals. Thus, for example, if a target is a transnational actor (such the United Nations or a United Nations organization), then it may need to be pressured by groups from around the world; in such a case, creating a network of transnational activists would make applying multiple sources of pressure a possibility. Finally, a third condition is when conferences and other international arenas provide spaces for such organization and network strengthening to occur.[6]

All three conditions have important applications to the global treatment access movement. Most of the governments of the world either currently or historically have failed to protect the rights of PWAs through violations of privacy and tolerance of discrimination—in education, housing, employment, and provision of medical services among others. Thus, it can be very useful for AIDS activists to reach beyond their borders to find citizens of other places to publicize conditions and pressure their governments to change policies. PWAs in the United States, for example, who remember, or even experienced, what it was like in the 1980s when HIV-positive people were refused treatment by hospital workers who feared contagion can now help to advocate against such treatment where it is still occurring. Similarly, the goal of universal treatment access has involved a multiplicity of targets, including governments of both developed and developing nations, transnational corporations, and transnational entities including the United Nations, the WTO, and the IMF and World Bank. In all these cases, transnational networking brings new talent and energy and bodies into the struggle. Finally, the development over the past twenty years of a different form of transnational network, the epistemic community of scientists, health care workers, and other professionals who work in the field of AIDS, has guaranteed the existence of regular international meetings and conferences that have become fertile grounds for international networking, media work, and the implementation of international campaigns.

Overall, Keck and Sikkink point out, a central, perhaps *the* central, task of social movements and by extension transnational advocacy networks is "*to make possible the previously unimaginable, by framing problems in such a way that their solution comes to appear inevitable.*"[7] This is precisely what the global treatment access movement has done. In the space of a few short years, access to ARVs has gone from an idea seldom discussed (and when it was discussed, always dismissed as utterly impractical) to a moral imperative embodied in UN-based declarations of commitment, international government organization plans, and even a U.S. president's State of the Union address. That global treatment access has been accepted as a goal by powerful actors originally dead-set against it is remarkable; that implementation of this goal is began in earnest in a political landscape hostile to any nonsecurity-based foreign policy initiatives is even more surprising. How this is happening, and how the global treatment access movement envisions its forward trajectory are the important issues that the second half of the book will seek to explain.

Such a discussion should be prefaced with an important caveat, however. This discussion is necessarily both incomplete and impossible to neatly compartmentalize. The primary goal of this book is to explore the development and operation of the *treatment access movement* which is contained as one movement within the larger AIDS activist movement. Even within this narrower movement, the cast of actors is very large, and beyond the scope of this book to fully catalog. Moreover, the situation is further complicated by the multifaceted issues prioritized by many of the groups prominent in the global treatment access movement. In the United States and within certain other countries there are a few organizations like Health GAP that have devoted themselves primarily to the goal of universal treatment access. Many of the organizations with which they work, however, do not have such an exclusive focus. Some, such as MSF, have an entirely different primary mission, and run specific campaigns for this particular cause. Others, such as some national groups like the Thai Drug Users Network, are organized around certain issues that must be resolved even before treatment can be meaningfully pursued. Thus, Health GAP has been chosen as a way of situating the discussion of these events for three reasons. First, it is an organization whose central purpose is global treatment access, which is the movement explored in this book. Second, it is an entirely U.S.-based organization, and it is the goal of this book to view what is actually a global movement from a U.S. perspective. Finally, within this movement, different organizations have played different, though equally important, roles. One of the most critical roles of Health GAP, often in conjunction with the ACT UP groups from which it drew much inspiration, most of its staff, and many of its volunteers, has been as a *catalyst*—especially in terms of finding and exploiting political fault lines or in the words of its staff, serving as the "crowbar in the crack" to open up new campaign opportunities.

This ability to see emerging opportunities and quickly act on them has been a signature skill of AIDS activism generally—so much so that the language describing its tactics, such as "zaps," reflects this. But in a global context, especially when working with broad coalitions and/or groups in developing countries with very different cultures and access to communications systems for group decision making, this can sometimes be more problematic. These complications have been issues not only for AIDS activists, but for transnational issue advocacy networks generally. In a piece broadly critical of the optimistic view of transnational networking put forward by Keck and Sikkink, Clifford Bob has argued that in fact, such networks can work at the expense of the organizations and individuals on the developing country side. He argues that not only does the need to find sympathetic (well-resourced) Western NGO "partners" create a tragic form of competition among non-Western groups, but also that it leads to the distortion of priorities and goals, in order to conform with the Western NGO missions. Further, he notes that often, these North-South NGO collaborations favor Southern organizations led by a single strong, charismatic leader. This is because the presence of such a leader eases the tasks of the Northern NGO, both in communicating with the group and in media relations where there can be a single spokesperson, and because the presence of multiple leaders may lead to internal strife that complicates these same tasks. Thus Western NGOs often contribute to a (sometimes unspoken) expectation of undemocratic and antiparticipatory organizational structure for developing country groups.[8]

This potential conflict of good intentions with operational realities is all the more poignant in the case of AIDS activism because a central tenet of AIDS organizing has always been the privileging of PWA self-empowerment. Thus, a crucial continuing challenge is finding a way to apply the strengths that have served the domestic AIDS movement so well to the much more complex and multifaceted global movement. The struggle to reconcile the successful legacy of domestic AIDS activism with the stark inequities inherent in every aspect of the global pandemic animates the treatment access campaigns described in the chapters that follow.

Chapter 3

Many Places, One Goal: Connecting Global Actors

"Those of us who live affluent lives, well attended by medical care and treatment should not ask how Germans or white South Africans could tolerate living in proximity to moral evil. We do so ourselves today, in proximity to the impending illness and death of many millions of people with AIDS. This will happen, unless we change the present government ineptitude and corporate blocking. Available treatments are denied to those who need them for the sake of aggregating corporate wealth for shareholders who by African standards are already unimaginably affluent."[1] With these powerful words, HIV-positive South African High Court Justice Edwin Cameron helped to set a very different tone for the 2000 International AIDS Conference than that of previous meetings. The speech he was giving was the newly instituted Jonathan Mann Memorial Lecture, and it was being given at the first International AIDS conference held in a city of a developing country—Durban, South Africa.

Cameron's words within the halls were a restatement of sentiments that had been aggressively promoted on the streets. On Sunday July 9, the opening day of the conference, some 5000 demonstrators, many of them wearing T-shirts proclaiming "HIV positive," took to the streets in a spirited protest demanding lower prices for lifesaving AIDS medicines. The theme of the 1998 Geneva meeting, "Bridging the Gap," was viewed cynically when it was spoken about in an abstract way on podiums by official leaders and presenters. But in 2000 the idea of treatment was embraced in earnest by activists both in and outside the conventional halls in Durban. The protest march was notable not only in demonstrating the ability of the South African AIDS activist Treatment Action Campaign (TAC) to mobilize thousands of grassroots activists from deeply impoverished affected townships; it also showcased the possibilities of collaborative work within the global treatment activist movement that had furnished organizations and individuals that had supported TAC in this project.

The Durban meeting would be followed by a remarkable string of opportunities and victories around the world, all occurring within a highly compressed time frame. On the opportunity front, 2001 would be the year that blew the possibilities of global ARV treatment wide open. First came the drastic dropping of prices of combination ARV therapy and then a UN-initiated Global Fund to fight the three largest infectious disease killers, to help developing nations access the newly affordable medications. The Indian generic drug company Cipla kicked off the year 2001 with an offer in early February to furnish a version of the combination therapy to the international medical relief organization MSF for $350 a year per patient. Cipla's announcement was actually all the more noteworthy because it was a major embarrassment to the brand-name pharmaceutical industry, which had with much fanfare unveiled unspecified major price reductions in May 2000. The subsequent country-by-country drug-by-drug working out of details meant that only two countries, Senegal and Uganda, had achieved any kind of price cut for triple therapy medications even six months after the deal was unveiled. Cipla's announcement, which severely undercut the best price deal reached in Senegal of $950 per year, set in motion a dynamic of competition that would result in the dropping of prices for combination ARV therapy from over $10,000 to less than $300 per year. In early April a vision for how greatly expanded treatment might happen was articulated in a consensus statement signed by more than one hundred Harvard faculty members, including noted economist Jeffrey Sachs. The statement envisioned the possibility of raising an emergency worldwide fund that could initially use $1.1 billion to treat a million Africans. A few weeks later at a meeting of the Organization of African Unity in Abuja, Nigeria, UN Secretary General Kofi Annan would reiterate the call for the creation of such a new fund which would become the Global Fund to Fight AIDS, Tuber-culosis, and Malaria (Global Fund). These openings in opportunity would be complemented by a series of country-specific battles waged against the branded pharmaceutical industry, which was the most intractable foe of widely available generic versions of antiretroviral combinations. In South Africa, in Brazil, and in Kenya, the industry would be dealt some serious blows, as well. All three countries would pass legislation or issue rulings making it easier to procure and/or use generic medications to treat their people. Perhaps even more damaging from the industry perspective, the actions of all three countries would occur under the close scrutiny of AIDS activists within the countries, and be amplified by the treatment activist network operating outside their borders. The cases would be different, but all three would be presented as morality plays in which the less powerful actors were taking the moral high road by promoting a right to health against stronger industries and governments pursuing crass material interests.

Taken together, these developments constitute a mutually reinforcing pattern between activist victories and new political opportunities. Some of these developments, such as Kenya's parliamentary victory against the drug industry, were superficially internal domestic issues; yet even in such cases, global pressure from transnational activist networks was applied, and the results had ramifications beyond the specific country. The introduction of affordable medicines, the dropping of legal actions against South Africa and Brazil by the pharmaceutical industry and the U.S. government respectively, and the call for the Global Fund all constituted major victories for activists who had been exerting pressure for exactly these results. They also created new opportunities for further activist goals and campaigns.

Another major hallmark of this time period (July 2000–June 2001), and of the developments that characterized it, was its increasingly global focus, in terms of targets and partners. The Gore zaps and subsequent targeting of the Bush administration were carried out by a group of U.S.-based activists targeting individuals within the U.S. government. As the campaign stepped up, American activists continued to place heavy emphasis on American targets, including the various actors within the U.S. government, and pharmaceutical companies and lobbyists based in the United States. But they expanded their targets to include international entities like United Nations agencies and the World Trade Organization, as well as multinational companies and lobbyists, largely but not exclusively pharmaceutical companies and their global lobbies. They also increasingly worked in partnership with both transnational nongovernment organizations, such as MSF and Oxfam, and with AIDS activists organizations in both developing and developed countries, such as TAC in South Africa and ACT UP Paris in France. And in a number of cases, such as the South African pharmaceutical battle and especially the Kenyan parliamentary struggle, American activism played a clearly supporting role to struggles going on within the borders of other countries.

This chapter picks up the story of the U.S.-based treatment access movement as it integrates itself into, and helps to shape, the rapidly developing transnational issue advocacy network that is the global treatment access movement. The emergence of this transnational movement is critical to the overall goal of expanded treatment access. Yet it also exposes weaknesses and challenges to the U.S.-based elements of the movement, which must find ways to organize and campaign effectively across the barriers of not only time and distance, but also race, class, culture, and vastly unequal distributions of resources between elements of the movement.

INTERNATIONAL LINKAGES IN THE AIDS ACTIVIST MOVEMENT

In a sense, Health GAP was always part of a transnational movement. There were transnational nongovernmental organizations, including MSF and the International Gay and Lesbian Human Rights Commission, present at its earliest meetings, and very important internationally linked actions, including protests at international meetings and internationally supported actions by domestic groups, have been features of AIDS activism for years. But certainly, the connections became much stronger as the work, and especially the victories, related to getting pills into bodies in developing countries began to accelerate. Given this major acceleration of organizing across international lines and subsequent victories, it is reasonable to situate the forging of a transnational issue advocacy network as beginning around the year 2000.

How U.S.-based treatment activists were able to work with other elements of the global movement to consolidate a genuine transnational advocacy network in the face of numerous internal and external obstacles is the central narrative of the remainder of this chapter. In an attempt to simplify a necessarily complex and near-infinite web of actors, the next section of the chapter will provide a brief overview and description of some of the major groups that have been particularly critical from the U.S. perspective in the network. From there, it will move to a narrative that describes some of the key events that occurred mostly within a one-year framework that allowed for the building and growth of the transnational network.

KEY COMPONENTS OF THE TRANSNATIONAL ADVOCACY NETWORK

The global arena of AIDS treatment activism within which Health GAP operates is very large and complex. Just as the political opportunity structure operating at the global level has shaped developments of the transnational advocacy network, so have individual structures and histories within countries and regions shaped the activist responses at the domestic and regional levels. Additionally, in some countries, there have been one or two organizations that have played critical roles in the global treatment activist movement, while in other countries, there are more complicated coalitions of actors. The linkages between these groups have come about in a variety of ways. In some cases, shared geography, such as the presence of U.S. offices of transnational organizations, has greatly facilitated face-to-face contact of people working in various groups. In other cases, contacts have been made, particularly at important international meetings such as international AIDS conferences, and then maintained via electronic communication—especially listservs, cell phones, and conference calls. Sometimes particular campaigns have also facilitated connections, as campaign coordinators have reached out to find new coalition members interested in the goals of specific initiatives. The following sections briefly outline some of the key network actors with which the U.S.-based movement has most frequently worked.

The Treatment Action Campaign of South Africa

Within the complex world of AIDS activism, one group that has achieved something approaching legendary status is the Treatment Action Campaign of South Africa. South Africa is home to a wide array of civil society–based organizations rooted in different communities and economic sectors that have done passionate and instrumental work on HIV/AIDS. The country-wide AIDS Consortium, for instance, notes on its Web site a membership of over 1,000 mainly community-based groups.[2] There are a number of prominent national organizations, such as the National Association of PWAs (NAPWA) and the AIDS Law Project, as well as groups from other sectors, that have played critical roles in important AIDS struggles, such as the Congress of South African Trade Unions (COSATU) and innumerable small local groups with few resources but important links to the communities they serve. But in terms of international recognition, leadership, and linkages, TAC holds a place of prominence not only in South Africa, but in the global treatment access movement.

The birth of the organization came on International Human Rights Day (December 10) 1998, when a group of about fifteen people gathered on the steps of Saint George's Cathedral in Cape Town, South Africa, to launch a new campaign under the auspices of NAPWA to demand medical treatment for people living with HIV. By the end of the day, the protestors had also gathered more than 1,000 signatures on a petition calling on the government to create a universal treatment plan for people living with HIV.

TAC eventually became independent of NAPWA and opened branches in other parts of the country. By 2004 it was reported to have 8,300 active members organized into 150 chapters around the country, all run by an executive committee elected during an annual membership meeting. According to a 2001 news story which characterized TAC as taking only two years to "march from nowhere to the front lines," even TAC's leadership did not expect it to grow so fast. The story notes that some 169 trade unions, NGOs, and faith-based organizations joined TAC's struggle after it was launched, supporting Secretary Mark Heywood's claim that TAC was "building as broad a front as possible, particularly for anyone who is pro-poor, pro-labour and pro-feminist."[3] In addition to campaigning for affordable HIV/AIDS treatments, TAC also explicitly works for treatment for pregnant women to prevent HIV transmission to newborns, advocates for a national health system that will provide equal treatment for all South Africans, and promotes treatment literacy and living and leadership skills for people with HIV.

Taking on these goals has meant targeting both the international brand-name pharmaceutical industry over patent rights and pricing of drugs and the South African government, which has famously questioned the efficacy and safety of AIDS drugs. In the mid-1990s it appeared that the government could be a source of leadership in the fight for access to affordable medications when it passed the Medicines Act that allowed for compulsory licensing and parallel importing. In fact, the subsequent fight with the brand-name pharmaceutical industry that resulted (and about which more is said later in this chapter) *did* serve as a rallying point for the international treatment access movement, which stood shoulder to shoulder with the South African government against the pharmaceutical corporations. In almost every other respect related to treatment, however, the South African government has not only failed to show leadership: it has been a shameful obstacle in the desperate struggle to get medicines to the people who need them.

In 1999 President Thabo Mbeki and Health Minister Manto Shabalala-Msimang both began to openly challenge the use of the antiretroviral AZT as treatment, and as a means of preventing the transmission of HIV from mother to child. By 2000, Mbeki was soliciting the ideas of AIDS denialists who argue that HIV does not cause AIDS and that AIDS medications are a dangerous scam. He convened a panel of these denialist together with other scientists to reexamine these questions and gave a speech at the 13th International AIDS Conference his country was hosting in Durban where he publicly questioned the link between HIV and AIDS once again. Six months later, after refusing to make AZT widely available at public hospitals to prevent mother-to-child transmission, the government lost in a High Court ruling that favored TAC and other activists and pediatricians by requiring universal access to the program.[4] After much struggle back and forth, the government would eventually announce plans to begin public treatment in 2003, but movement would continue to be painfully slow and wrought with continued mixed messages from the minister of health about the dangers of the drugs.

TAC's support includes notable individual figures like Nelson Mandela, as well as COSATU, the South African NGO coalition (SANGOCO), and major religious organizations. TAC's best-known asset, however, is its charismatic chairman, Zackie Achmat. Referred to as "the Gandhi of the AIDS movement," Achmat became internationally known for his refusal to access through private means antiretroviral medications until they were distributed by the South African government to all of his fellow PWAs. He formally abandoned this pledge, to the great relief of fellow activists worldwide, on August 4, 2003, when the government announced its intention to begin distributing antiretrovirals through public clinics. During his boycott Achmat suffered the same dangerous and painful ailments as his fellow South Africans with AIDS, including life-threatening lung infections. His public pledge compounded his personal trials by stripping him of his privacy as the global AIDS community collectively held its breath with each new missive of his failing health. It also opened him up to criticism from a variety of quarters—from the government with which he had once been closely allied and with whom he had struggled for years during Apartheid, and from individuals throughout the world who challenged his choices, arguing he was of greater use to the movement as a physically healthy leader within it. But his refusal to take the drugs that could keep him healthy, together with his leadership at rallies and protests and well-publicized participation in media events like the open smuggling of generic drugs from Thailand, have made him not only a leader but also a powerful symbol in the struggle for AIDS treatment.

According to McAdam's political process model, the organizational strength of a movement is predicated in part on membership, which is often drawn from preexisting struggles and movements. This is certainly true in the case of TAC, whose leadership as well as much of its rank-and-file membership was heavily involved in the earlier anti-Apartheid struggle. These earlier experiences have been critical as well in providing previous experience with the extremely useful tactic of what Petchesky has called the "proactive use of law," using litigation as a means of providing a connection between law, human rights, and direct action.[5] Two of TAC's greatest victories have come using the courts to pressure first a transnational target (the international pharmaceutical industry) and then a domestic target (the executive branch of its own government). Along the way it has skillfully made use of not only the final outcomes, but also the process itself to continuously build coalitions and support for both the battle at hand and the larger movement of which these milestones are markers.

GAPA, Grupo Pela VIDDA and the Brazilian State

Although Brazil and South Africa are home to what are probably the most well-known AIDS social movements within the developing world, organizationally speaking, they are very different. South African activism has become world famous in large part because of the leadership of a particular organization, and especially one of its leaders. Additionally, much of its work is focused internally, targeting its own government, which has been famously reluctant to provide access to antiretroviral medications. This stands in stark contrast to the other highly publicized AIDS activist success story, Brazil. The Brazilian case exemplifies a wholly different model of mobilization in the face of a health crisis, with remarkable integration between government officials, particularly from within the Ministry of Health, and elements of civil society organizations and activists from, among others, gay rights organizations, AIDS service and activist groups, and women's organizations.

Two structural elements have facilitated the initial civil society demands and subsequent favorable government responses within Brazil. These were the federal system under which the Brazilian government is organized and the earlier successful incorporation of health care as a human right in the 1988 Brazilian constitution promoted by the so-called sanitary movement. As in the United States, the response to AIDS began at the local level, most notably in São Paulo, which was both the center of an emerging gay liberation movement and the site of most of the early reported AIDS cases. There, gay activists began meeting with the State Secretariat of Health as early as 1983, which formed a working group on AIDS in mid-1983 within the Division of Hansen's Disease and Sanitary Dermatology.[6] This working group would become the foundation for the State AIDS Program, which would in turn serve as a model for other states in the country so that, by 1985, when the National Ministry of Health began work on a National AIDS Program, at least eleven states and federal districts (of twenty-seven) already had state AIDS programs in place.[7]

Of course, like the original program in São Paulo, these state-based programs and the national one have not arisen in a vacuum. They have been established in response to a flourishing civil society movement with many organizational members. Three of the most well known of these are the locally based chapters of Support Group for AIDS Prevention (GAPA), beginning with GAPA-São Paulo, the Brazilian Interdisciplinary AIDS

Association (ABIA) founded in Rio de Janeiro in 1986, and the Grupo Pela VIDDA-Rio de Janeiro, which began as a project within ABIA and now maintains chapters in a number of cities throughout Brazil. Although all three organizations have worked at the policy level, advocating for progressive programs of prevention and treatment, GAPA was at least initially more locally focused, while ABIA was always more nationally oriented. Two of the most influential early leaders of these organizations, and of the AIDS movement generally, were the "two Herberts"—Herbert de Souza (more popularly known as Betinho) and Herbert Daniel. Both men had been progressive political exiles and then were active in the redemocratization efforts in the 1980s upon their respective returns. Betinho, a hemophiliac whose two brothers were also HIV positive, is credited with providing the impetus for ABIA, while Daniel became the founder and first president of Grupo Pela VIDDA-Rio de Janeiro, the first explicit organization of people living with HIV/AIDS in the country.

These organizations, though possibly the most influential, are certainly not isolated. Rather, they have worked in tandem with numerous other groups drawn from various sectors of civil society. Parker notes as early as 1990 that the 2nd National Meeting of AIDS NGOs had representation of thirty-eight groups including the Religious Support Group Against AIDS (ARCA) from the ecumenical Institute of Religious Studies (ISER), and organizations representing both gay and sex worker rights.[8] And, as women became increasingly affected, organizations representing feminist, lesbian, and popular health concerns have joined the movement in growing numbers.

The interaction between civil society and government in Brazil has been exceptional, particularly in the sense that Brazilian AIDS activists appear to have been able to avoid the trap of co-optation, and the subsequent de-radicalization of the movement. Petchesky has noted that a key difference in the Brazilian case "is the responsiveness of government officials, particularly in the national, state and municipal health departments, to popular and NGO demands." She further notes that this is not coincidental "since many of these officials, especially at middle-bureaucratic and municipal levels, have come out of the gay, lesbian and feminist movements."[9] At the same time as the government has been remarkably receptive to advocacy networks, the activists and advocacy organizations have managed to maintain their independence. For example, in the early 1990s, AIDS NGO leadership prominently called for impeachment hearings of the Collor government on corruption charges.[10]

Perhaps the key dynamic to consider in analyzing the Brazilian case is that, after making the critical decisions to push forward with proactive and visionary policy initiatives on the prevention and, especially, the treatment fronts, in the middle and late 1990s, the Brazilian government had *itself* become an activist actor on the world stage. By the year 2000, it had moved from being primarily a target for Brazilian activists to an active participant in the international treatment activist movement. It had shown that it was possible to defy the collective wisdom of the World Bank, the multinational brand-name pharmaceutical industry, and the United States. For various reasons, all of these entities had been opposed to Brazil's decision to pay for a universal treatment access program, and to produce the medications in it. Although the World Bank would eventually come around to the Brazilian idea that treatment could be cost-effective, the brand-name industry and the U.S. government that supported it would continue to fear Brazil's patent-breaking potential. Yet, just like the nonstate activist groups with which it allied, Brazil has been able to take its case to the global court of public opinion and mount convincing arguments that it is operating from the morally superior (as well as cost-effective) position.

The Agua Buena Human Rights Association

Because Brazil, together with the Brazilian organizations that have pushed its progressive policies, has been such a leader, it is easy for the hundreds of other organizations doing treatment access work to be overshadowed. Among the many AIDS advocacy organizations pressing for the rights of PWAs, one of the most active in the treatment access movement is the Costa Rica–based Agua Buena Human Rights Association. This group was founded in 1997 by psychologist Richard Stern, who was born in the United States but has lived in Costa Rica for fifteen years. His inspiration came from attendance at the 1996 International AIDS Conference that trumpeted the success of combination antiretroviral therapy. Returning to San Jose, Stern helped to promote a Supreme Court case that won the right to treatment for Costa Ricans living with HIV; he and his organization then turned their attention to treatment access in other parts of the region, including Guatemala, Honduras, El Salvador, Panama, Nicaragua, Belize, Peru, Bolivia, Ecuador, Jamaica, the Dominican Republic, St. Lucia, and Paraguay.[11]

Although it is a very small organization run by Stern and a handful of staff, it has been a very important voice for treatment access in the under-represented areas of Latin America (with the significant exception of Brazil) and the Caribbean. Stern and his organization actively challenge not only the U.S., Latin American, and Caribbean governments, but also UN organizations including UNAIDS and the Pan-American Health

Organization (PAHO), individual drug companies, and other organizations within the AIDS and treatment access movements. Often the focus of these challenges is different than that of organizations like Health GAP, which tend to concentrate on large demands for starting new programs and ramping up their financial support. Many of Agua Buena's campaigns have pushed existing programs to implement their services, particularly for treatment, faster and more completely.

The Kenya Coalition for Access to Essential Medicines

Although sub-Saharan Africa is the most heavily impacted region in the world, activists organizations face severe mobilization obstacles. The region is also the poorest in the world, and many of the people who are most severely affected by HIV/AIDS are so deeply challenged by the connected horrors of grinding poverty and untreated HIV complications that organizing becomes a luxury. Where organizing has been most successful, one of the important tools has been the use of coalitions which allow groups with possibly impoverished grassroots memberships to work in conjunction with organizations which may have greater resources, skills, and outside connections, but less local knowledge and experience. One such coalition is the Kenya Coalition for Access to Essential Medicines. Made up of fifteen national and international NGOs, its membership includes large organizations broadly supporting goals on development (such as Action Aid), international health (groups like Health Action International, MSF and Pharmaciens sans Frontières). It also includes Kenyan professional groups (such as the International Federation of Women Lawyers-Kenya and the Kenyan Medical Association) and Kenyan AIDS-specific groups including Women Fighting AIDS in Kenya, Society for Women and AIDS in Kenya, and Nyumbani (a famous AIDS orphanage outside of Nairobi). The group was formed following a meeting initiated by MSF.

The Kenya Coalition has a number of strengths which it has used to good effect. These include a diversity of skills within its membership because of the varied partners within the coalition; access to resources and press outside the country, particularly because of international NGOs within the coalition; and its home location in Nairobi, which is not only the capital of Kenya, but also a regional base of operation for the United Nations and many Western donor groups and international NGOs. The coalition was active in pressing the parliament for a drug bill similar to an earlier controversial one passed in South Africa, as well as in conducting campaigns directed to the media and the public at large on access to AIDS drugs.

The Kenya Coalition has been an important actor in the still-larger Pan African HIV/AIDS Treatment Access Movement (PATAM) inaugurated in August 2002 in Cape Town, South Africa, by leading activist cofounders Zackie Achmat of TAC and Milly Katana, lobbying and advocacy officer of the Health Rights Action Group in Uganda. Like ACT UP, PATAM has no paid staff, no office, and explicitly puts PWAs at the center of the movement. It is a loose network that coordinates its activities through a Steering Committee composed of representatives from the regions of North, West, East, southern and Central Africa.

Thai AIDS Treatment Action Group (TTAG), Thai Drug Users Network (TDN), and Thai Network of People Living with HIV/AIDS (TNP+)

Despite the nearc-exclusive focus by Health GAP and other organizations on AIDS treatment, many close allies have broader goals. National organizations necessarily respond to the demographics and needs of their memberships and constituencies, and in Thailand, one of the most dramatic needs is among the injection drug using community. Although Thailand has been hailed globally as a success story in bringing down its transmission rates among those engaging in sexual risk behaviors, not all high-risk groups have fared as well. The pragmatic harm reduction approach taken in its "100% condom use" prevention programs among commercial sex workers has not been applied to injection drug users. In fact, in February 2001, when Prime Minister Thaksin Shinawatra assumed office, he announced that fighting illegal drug use would be a top priority, and in January 2003 called for a war on drugs which would include very extreme measures— including the summary execution of suspected drug dealers. Although initially the country supported the announced crackdown, which is directed at the country's methamphetamine problem, the citizenry has since reversed its position as more and more innocent bystanders have been killed. In a three month period more than 2,000 "alleged drug suspects," including children, were killed.[12]

In the face of such draconian measures, the Thai activist movement was forced to respond, which it did in several pathbreaking ways. Previous work by Thai activists had revolved around promoting the manufacture of generic antiretroviral medication, beginning with a high-profile case involving the manufacture of didanosine, a drug patented by Bristol-Myers Squibb, and pressing the Thai government to provide a national treatment plan. But the new government war against drug users forced treatment activists to emphasize that treatment accessibility was a farce when roughly a third of those needing treatment were literally hiding from the government that was supposed to be providing it.

The Thai situation provides a good example of the way that existing groups can not only work together, but also help to establish new groups that promote complementary, but different goals. Here, two of the most important groups working on treatment access, the Thai Network of People Living with HIV/AIDS (TNP+) and the Thai AIDS Treatment Action Group (TTAG), facilitated the rise of a third group, the Thai Drug Users Network (TDN). TNP+ was a relatively well-established group, founded in 1996, a year after Thai PWAs had been given an opportunity to come together to strategize at a 1995 Asia/Pacific Islands regional AIDS conference in Chiang Mai. It had taken on a mandate to support PWAs, promote their human rights and welfare, and cooperate with NGOs and government in working to end the epidemic.[13] TTAG was established in 2002, with the support of two outside NGOs, MSF and the American Jewish World Service Committee. Its mission adds advocating for the right to AIDS treatment to other goals which are similar to those of TNP+. Preexisting organizational structures, membership, and especially leadership were instrumental in helping this third organization get off the ground quickly. Both the Director, Paisan Tan-Ud, and the International Advocacy Coordinator, Karyn Kaplan (an American founding volunteer with Health GAP and former staff member of IGLHRC), of TTAG, for example, helped provide critical leadership to TDN in charting its inaugural path. Paisan had also been a leader in other organizations, notably serving as founding chair of TNP+ for five years.

In the face of an extremely hostile environment, TDN was able to make excellent use of several openings in the domestic and global political structure. The first of these occurred when TDN became the first nongovernmental organization ever to successfully apply to the Global Fund to AIDS, Tuberculosis, and Malaria. The Global Fund, mentioned earlier in this chapter as another of the pivotal developments of 2001, was set up to allow countries to apply competitively for grants to combat the three major infectious disease killers. But a requirement was that country grants be the product of Country Coordinating Mechanisms (CCMs), which were supposed to be representative of major stakeholders within the country. TDN successfully argued that, given the deeply antagonistic and, in fact, deadly disposition of its government, it could not reasonably be expected to be represented fairly within the CCM process. In addition to the landmark Global Fund grant (which was also very important to the global treatment access and larger AIDS activist movements in setting a precedent for direct civil society funding), TDN and the other Thai activist groups also took advantage of the decision to situate the 15th International AIDS Conference that occurred in July 2004 to work with other treatment activists and AIDS activists generally, to publicize the plight of drug users in Thailand through demonstrations, meetings, and media work throughout the conference.

Partners in the Global North: MSF and ACT UP Paris

An important characteristic of the treatment access movement is that it has network organizations from both the global North and South. Two of the most prominent non-U.S. Northern NGOs in the movement, MSF and ACT UP Paris, share a commitment to the goal of universal treatment access and have their roots in France. They are very different organizations, however. MSF is actually an international NGO, with health care professional volunteers from around the world. It is by far the larger of the two, has a much broader mission, is older (having been founded in 1971), and has much wider name recognition. Its overall mission is to provide medical aid wherever it is needed throughout the world, and to raise awareness of the conditions of those it serve is. It is a very well-known group, and has an international reputation as the "first in, last out" in providing services in war zones and other highly dangerous situations. It has over 500 medical programs in 80 countries. Winner of the 2000 Nobel Peace Prize, MSF's involvement in universal AIDS treatment access is part of a larger project entitled the Access to Essential Medicines Campaign which began in 1999. The project seeks to provide affordable treatment for a variety of illnesses that affect poor people throughout the world. Its advocacy work is aided by its field work, which includes a number of well-known sites around the world that were among the first to demonstrate that antiretroviral treatment could be effectively administered in very resource-poor settings with compliance rates at or above those found in developed countries. MSF's relatively large size and ability to specialize in both advocacy and on-the-ground treatment afford it and the movement it supports interesting advantages. Not only are the on-the-ground sites sources of valuable information for activists to disseminate, as in the case cited above about treatment efficacy, but these locally based professionals are often themselves part of local activist organizations and coalitions, or offer critical support in their founding. For instance, MSF works very closely with TAC in South Africa, both on political campaigns and more recently in an actual treatment program being jointly run by the two groups. It has provided both membership and direction to the Kenya Coalition for Access to Essential

Medicines, and it, together with the American Jewish World Service, helped to found TTAG in Thailand.

In contrast to the extensive reach and on-the-ground programming of MSF, ACT UP Paris is much more similar to the other surviving chapters of ACT UP in the United States. Like the other ACT UP chapters, it is locally based, drew its original strength from, and maintains continuing association with, the gay community, and initially focused on domestic issues before broadening to an international treatment agenda. The transition from a domestic to an international focus was relatively late in its history. Also like the other ACT UP chapters, it is an explicitly activist organization, combining demonstrations and direct action tactics with sophisticated policy analysis. And like the other chapters, it maintains its independence from government and the pharmaceutical industries by refusing funding from either. However, in contrast to ACT UP New York and Philadelphia, which have maintained an all-volunteer membership and leadership, since 1996 ACT UP Paris has had paid staffers (currently nine, although some are part time) and has differentiated work roles accordingly. ACT UP Paris also has about twenty to twenty-five volunteer members who work in the office, as well as weekly meetings that draw about fifty people. ACT UP Paris began to work on the issue of global treatment access long before Health GAP came into existence, back in 1992, and accelerated its work on the topic after 1996 when the positive effects of HAART became widely known.[14]

Although, as noted above, the groups listed here represent only a sample within a much larger patchwork of interconnected organizations and networks, their descriptions help to show the diversity of the movement. There are organizations working for treatment access around the globe, in both developed and developing countries. Some, like MSF, are large and, by NGO standards, relatively old. Even older and more established than MSF is Oxfam, a British-based antipoverty agency working in over seventy countries that was founded in the 1940s as a famine relief organization. Like MSF, and a number of other INGOs, Oxfam has added AIDS to its portfolio in recent years. Oxfam has also been particularly active on treatment access, especially in fighting the intellectual property laws that keep drugs inaccessible in developing countries. Recognizing HIV for the global health and development priority it is, it has been added as a key component to its missions. Others, like the Kenya Coalition for Access to Essential Medicines, are loose affiliations of other organizations that have come together to pursue a common interest. Still others, like TAC, are mass-based organizations that have become not only models for AIDS organizing, but also an example of successful civil society activity generally.

Although practice does not always mirror principle, all the organizations highlighted here have several other commonalities that are broadly shared among almost all the players within the transnational network advocating for global treatment access. The network is guided by a human rights framework that privileges the right to health over the right to profits and values all people equally (though this second point has at times been challenged by groups allied with the treatment access movement, who have charged that treatment activists have occasionally privileged the relatively less controversial arguments for treatment over other equity and antidiscrimination work on behalf of marginalized populations). This framework also means that they simultaneously work for the rights of PLWHAs and recognize the importance of their representation and leadership within their organizations. All are dedicated to nonviolent tactics, and most support in principle (though it may be too dangerous for themselves to practice) disruptive protest as a potential tool. The fact that the organizations cover a wide spectrum of forms and sizes is often advantageous. On the smaller, more radical end some, like Health GAP and the ACT UP chapters, have the flexibility and speed to quickly identify opportunities and plan actions and campaigns to exploit them. But being allied with large NGOs with considerably more clout, name recognition, and resources means that these can be shared to help sustain campaigns and provide legitimacy of the cause to outsiders. Of course, these differences can also be the source of friction when competing ideas about the priority of a particular campaign or tactic come into play. But usually, the shared sensibilities identified above form a values-based glue that holds together the transnational movement in the face of powerful governments and corporations who are their primary opponents, and allows members of the network to come back together even in the case of friction within a given campaign.

PIGGYBACKING ON HISTORY: PIVOTAL EVENTS AND OPPORTUNITIES FOR ORGANIZING

As noted previously, Keck and Sikkink suggest that transnational advocacy networks are most likely to occur under three conditions: when domestic activists are blocked from their targets and work with outside allies to apply external pressure, when activists believe that networks are a good way to reach their goals, and when conferences and international meetings provide space for connecting and reinforcing linkages. Although all three of these conditions have certainly been applied at various times and places within the global treatment access movement, much of the activity during the transnational advocacy network's formative period was made possible, or at least greatly facilitated by, several major international meetings held during this period. The first of these was the 13th International AIDS Conference held in Durban, South Africa.

The 13th conference was the first to be held in a developing country. In retrospect, it would have been hard to have picked a more critical place for the conference from the perspective of transnational advocacy networking. Not only was South Africa at the time carrying the largest burden of HIV/AIDS in the world, with an estimated four million people living with HIV, but those same people were facing a double obstacle to treatment. One problem was internal—a government that publicly questioned the causal link between HIV and AIDS—and the second was external—the combined force of United States and the international pharmaceutical industry attempting to pressure South Africa not to pursue the procurement of cheap drugs through the South African Medicines and Regulatory Devices Act discussed in Chapter 2. If ever there were a target-rich environment for treatment activism, this was it.

Seeing the opportunity and potential of the meeting for highlighting the cause of universal treatment access, TAC, together with allies like Health GAP, MSF, ACT UP Paris, and other NGOs within the treatment activist network, had prepared in advance. Western groups, including MSF and Health GAP, had helped with financial assistance as well as logistical support to on-the-ground organizing. Key members of the network also laid the groundwork by providing critical information at a time when they knew that the media and national governments were especially attuned to global HIV/AIDS stories and policy options. Prior to the conference's beginning, for instance, ACT UP Paris convened a meeting of governments of developing countries and generic drug manufacturers designed to highlight the options potentially available for providing affordable drugs. On the first day of the conference, MSF released a paper highlighting the feasibility of drastically cutting the prices of AIDS medications in the developing world. And during the conference various academic allies, including well-known economist Jeffrey Sachs and Partners in Health founder physician Paul Farmer, delivered presentations on the feasibility of mobilizing global resources for fighting global epidemic disease and of delivering antiretroviral treatment in resource-poor settings.

But the most visible sign of activism was certainly the protest march itself. TAC and its allies were able to mobilize more than 5,000 people, including members of South African labor unions, religious groups, and gay and lesbian organizations, to take part in the Global March for Treatment Access. The march not only became one of the major headlining events of the entire conference, but also served as a politicizing event for many of the people who took part in it. Pauline Ngunjiri, a Kenyan who had attended the conference as a journalist, would later become the codirector of the Society for Women and AIDS in Kenya (SWAK) and an active member of the Kenyan Coalition on Access to Essential Drugs. Through concerted activism, these and other Kenyan and international NGOs successfully pushed for the 2001 adoption of a Kenyan law similar to South Africa's. Ngunjiri has attributed her conversion from observer to activist to her participation in the South African protest when she "realized there was activism in the world" after agreeing to don a T-shirt, carry a banner, and march, rather than merely cover the event. Afterwards, she went on to become a leader in the Kenyan treatment activist movement.[15]

Following the excitement generated first by the call for affordable treatment in Durban and then the actual offer by Cipla CEO Yusuf Hamied of a $350 AIDS cocktail (a 96.6 percent discount of the same combination available in the United States for $10,400), attention shifted in large part to specific countries where battles were raging between activists and the multinational pharmaceutical industry. The most prominent of these in the press was a court fight in South Africa, in support of which a March 5 Global Day of Action was organized. Activists sought to support the South African government and to oppose the international drug companies who had brought a suit against the South African law that activists had faulted Gore for opposing. The controversy dated back to February 1998, when the Pharmaceutical Manufacturers Association (PMA)—the international lobby of the brand-new pharmaceutical companies, analogous to PhRMA in the United States—and thirty-nine drug companies had filed suit against the law. The suit dragged on for nearly three years and finally began in Pretoria on March 5. Timed to coincide with the opening of the case, TAC called for a Global Day of Action for solidarity actions and protests around the world. Protests were scheduled before and during the Global Day of Action in countries including Australia, Brazil, Canada, France, Germany, Great Britain, Italy, the Philippines, Thailand and, of course, the United States and South Africa.

In the United States, Health GAP member organizations ACT UP New York and ACT UP Philadelphia coordinated protests in New York City (at the offices of GlaxoSmithKline and Bristol-Myers Squibb, both on Park Avenue), in Philadelphia (at the GlaxoSmithKline headquarters), and in Washington DC (in a march extending from Bristol-Myers Squibb's offices to the White House to the offices of PhRMA). Additional protests were held in Boston and Berkeley, California.

Some of these protests, incidentally, carried significant potential risks to those involved. The February 20 protest at the New York City

GlaxoSmithKline offices resulted in arrest and subsequent felony charges for five activists ("the Glaxo five"). The charges were eventually dropped after a drawn-out court process over a year later. But in the interim TAC, and its high-profile leader Zackie Achmat, supported the Americans in a letter addressed to the district attorney, arguing that "it is not the five activists who should be on trial but the executives of GlaxoSmithKline and other pharmaceutical companies whose pricing policies and profiteering have led to the loss of thousands of lives" and promising that "TAC and our allies will mobilize support for the activists should you pursue these charges."

Back in South Africa on March 6, TAC scored a tactical victory when it was named by the High Court as a "friend of the court" (*amicus curiae*) empowered to speak on behalf of people living HIV/AIDS during the trial. The PMA, which had strenuously attempted to block TAC's application for this status, then tried to delay the trial a further four months to respond to this new development. The court granted a smaller period of time, agreeing to wait to reopen the trial on April 18.

In an attempt to quell what was rapidly becoming a public relations disaster, the drug industry spent much of the interlude making offers of price cuts of up to 90 percent to a number of African countries, including South Africa, as well as some offers of conditional drug donations; they then argued that the failure of South Africa to accept its offers constituted an unwillingness to resolve the issue. Of course, TAC and its allies across the globe, including Oxfam and MSF, as well as Health GAP and a host of other organizations and high-profile individuals, regarded such offers with skepticism. They noted among other objections that even the steep discounts did not bring the prices to the level of generics, that the donation programs came with too many strings, and that in any case, donations were rarely sustained on a long-term basis by donor corporations. For their part, they continued to ply the media with a picture of a greedy pharmaceutical industry intent on keeping dying people from accessing the medications they needed. Statements like that of Nelson Mandela, who argued that "the pharmaceuticals are exploiting the situation that exists in countries like South Africa" for which they "must be condemned," only added to the activists' momentum.[16]

The work paid off when on April 19, the day after the case reopened, the PMA and the pharmaceutical companies decided to cut their negative publicity losses, dropped the case, and agreed to pay the South African government's legal costs. Industry analysts termed the case a "public relations disaster" for the drug companies, and even company leadership conceded, in the words of GlaxoSmithKline Chief Executive J.P. Garnier, that

"We don't exist in a vacuum" and that "public opinion" was "a factor in our decision-making."[17]

One of the most important outcomes of the activist victory in South Africa was in the bounce it gave the treatment access movement. Internally and externally, it advertised the activist network's efficacy, or what McAdam refers to as cognitive liberation—the idea that people actually have the power to change an unjust situation. In other words, on April 20, the newspapers—in South Africa, in the United States, and indeed in countries around the world—were reporting that the massive pharmaceutical industry had been significantly and publicly defeated by an opposition force which brandished as its greatest weapon the power of persuasion. One of the places where activists were able to capitalize on this gain was Kenya, where, as a story title in the British medical journal *The Lancet* noted, "Generic drugs battle moves from South Africa to Kenya."[18]

In the Kenyan battle, the lines were similar to those drawn in South Africa. On one side were treatment activists, mainly from the Kenya Coalition on Access to Essential Medicines described in the previous section; on the other, the brand-name pharmaceutical industry. Unlike in South Africa, however, where the issue had already been passed as law and was being contested in the courts, the Kenyan fight played itself out with both sides targeting the Kenyan parliament, which had to decide the content of the Kenya Industrial Property Bill, and whether to pass it.

As in South Africa, with potentially damaging legislation looming on the horizon, the brand-name companies announced major price cuts. And, as in South Africa, activists rejected the announcements, again arguing that they were both insufficient and unsustainable. Price cuts without generic competition inherently exist at the whim of the manufacturer, who can withdraw them as soon as a particular political threat (in this case the pending legislation) has subsided. The Kenya Coalition was able to utilize the various talents of its members, organizing demonstrations, as well as gathering a petition with 50,000 Kenyan signatures in just five days. Perhaps most crucially, the Kenya Coalition also made excellent use of the press, particularly in embarrassing both the pharmaceutical industry and members of parliament, when it was able to expose a heavy-handed "lobbying" effort of the industry involving the financing of an all-expense-paid trip to a coastal resort for parliamentarians in order to discuss "compromise" legislation. On June 12, 2001, the Industrial Properties Bill was passed unanim-ously. Unfortunately, for the cause of treatment access, some months later the Kenyan government would announce that the importation of generic drugs it had enabled would still be blocked by WTO agreements.[19]

Thus, the Kenyan struggle over the Industrial Properties Bill was illustrative in several ways. On the one hand, it proved the ability of an internally mobilized coalition to use the power of persuasion, in this case, heavily backed by the power of information politics in the form of bad publicity for both the pharmaceutical industry and members of parliament, to achieve a seemingly improbable political end. It was a classic "boomerang" along the lines of the Keck and Sikkink model, allowing domestic activists to strengthen their hand by getting the word out outside their borders to create external pressure as well. On the other hand, the ultimate outcome, Kenyan capitulation to the brand–name industry in trade agreements illustrates both the multifaceted dimensions of power available to industry, and the need for activists to be vigilant at the multinational and binational fronts where these agreements are made.

FORWARD MOMENTUM IN BRAZIL

Throughout the struggles unfolding in Africa, one Latin American country was hosting its own ongoing battles with the pharmaceutical industry, and with the industry's most dogged defender, the U.S. government. The nation of Brazil, which had distinguished itself for both its aggressive prevention campaigns and its universal treatment access program, simultaneously drew praise and fire from the around the globe during 2001. The new year ushered in an extensive and widely read article by Tina Rosenberg that appeared in January in *The New York Times Magazine*. Full of praise for Brazil's accomplishments, the article vividly described the national treatment program, including Brazil's policy of manufacturing generic versions of several AIDS medications. Given this favorable publicity, as well as the decidedly negative press the drug companies were receiving because of the South African case, Brazil was in an excellent public relations position to press the pharmaceutical companies for price reductions on those branded drugs which it did not manufacture as generics. When Merck failed to negotiate a sufficient price cut on two drugs, Brazil began the development of a generic version of one of them, a product known as Stocrin (or generically, efavirenz), in a government-run laboratory. In late March, Merck gave in to the pressure and offered the drugs at $920 and $1,029 per year per patient (which was still higher than the price it offered in some other developing countries, but much lower than the U.S. price).

Although Merck had given in, that was hardly the end of the story. The U.S. government lodged a complaint against Brazil with the World Trade Organization, and a second drug company, Swiss-based Hoffman-La Roche, continued to hold out in its price negotiations. With support from global activists, and particularly U.S.-based activists including Health GAP who demonstrated outside the U.S. Trade Representative's Office and met with officials from the Brazilian consulate and the press in San Francisco to defend Brazil's actions, key members of the Brazilian government, including Health Minister Serra and President Cardoso himself, publicly refused to bow to U.S. pressure. Ultimately, in the spotlight of the impending United Nations Special Session on HIV/AIDS held in New York City, it was the United States that blinked. On the eve of the opening of the session, the U.S. government announced it had withdrawn its complaint and would resolve the issue with Brazil through bilateral negotiations. Although it did not offer a detailed explanation, news articles tended to note three things: the timing of the U.S. de-escalation, the embarrassment suffered by the pharmaceutical industry for having vigorously pursued the South Africa lawsuit that it ultimately abandoned, and the face-saving measure agreed to by Brazil that it would "consult" with the United States in the future.[20] Several months later, with no resolution with Roche in sight, Brazil took on a tough negotiating stance, once again threatening to begin manufacturing nelfinavir, the generic version of Roche's Viracept. To keep the Brazilian government from following through with its threats, Roche cut its price by a further 40 percent to the relief of the pharmaceutical industry and the disappointment of AIDS activists who were hoping for the precedent-setting issuance of a compulsory license that would have enabled Brazil to begin its manufacturing of the drug.

Despite the disappointment over Brazil's decision not to pursue a compulsory license, the cumulative effect of Brazil's actions was far-reaching. Brazil demonstrated that it was possible for a developing country to question both the trade position of the U.S. government and the pricing practices of the major pharmaceutical companies. Equally important, it demonstrated that the value of global public opinion was a formidable weapon, and that a framing of issues that pits human rights against the right to reap profits, and that privileges the former over the latter, has strong resonance in the court of public opinion.

PULLING THE PIECES TOGETHER: THE UNITED NATIONS MEETING ON AIDS

The time period that had opened up with the Durban meeting and expanded into the country-specific struggles outlined above concluded in late June in New York City at the three-day United Nations General Assembly Special Session (UNGASS) meeting, the first time ever that the

United Nations held a special session devoted to a disease. The purpose of the meeting was to bring together the nations of the world to draw up a single Declaration of Commitment which they would sign and which would serve as a blueprint for charting the future fight against the global pandemic. As with other special sessions, premeetings were held for months before to allow country delegations to wrangle over the wording of the document so that during the meeting there would be a draft to be finalized. At the behest of advocates, a key part of this Declaration was to be time-specific goals, allowing the world to have benchmarks for measuring progress for everything from women's empowerment to decreases in transmission rates within certain target populations to global treatment access.

Another key element of the meeting was the scheduling of four formal roundtable discussions meant to cover a variety of critical AIDS issue areas, in addition to dozens of "side events" that were scheduled within and nearby the UN building. The roundtable most directly relevant to AIDS treatment activists was roundtable 1, "HIV Prevention and Care." Round-table 2 was on "HIV/AIDS and Human Rights," Roundtable 3 dealt with "Socioeconomic Impacts," and Roundtable 4 covered "International Funding and Cooperation." Every organization that had been given accreditation was allowed a delegation of up to four people inside the UN (and some additional activists were able to gain access by applying for press credentials). The wide diversity of topics being covered at the roundtables and the UNGASS side events, together with the fact that it was being hosted in New York City, guaranteed an enormous civil society presence. Most of the organizations and activists explicitly involved up to this point in the U.S. treatment access movement were there, as well as many of the allied groups working on other aspects of AIDS issues. Attendees ranged from those working from a broader development advocacy, such as RESULTS and Global Exchange, to groups addressing several overlapping major AIDS issues, such as the Global AIDS Alliance and the African Services Committee. There were organizations that had started with very local roots but had developed an international focus, such as the Gay Men's Health Crisis, and groups with highly focused agendas, such as the International AIDS Vaccine Initiative and the Global Alliance for Vaccines and Immunizations. Some, such as MSF and Partners in Health, were eager to share their experience from the field, while a few, such as the philanthropic Soros Foundation, which funds prevention activities, especially needle exchange, sought to share their approaches. Representing the smallest tip of the proverbial iceberg, the groups mentioned here and dozens of others were drawn to the meeting as it presented a unique opportunity to meet with activist colleagues from around the world and get close to key policymakers to advocate for their issues.

As with the Durban International AIDS Conference, the UNGASS meeting began with a protest march. Repeating the slogan "Donate the dollars, drop the debt, treat the people, save the lives," thousands of marchers gathered under cloudy skies in New York City on June 23, 2001. The participants who walked the long route from their opening rally in Washington Square Park to the closing one thirty-five blocks north in Bryant Park represented a diversity of interests and nationalities. One news story covering the march noted participation from, among others, the Student Global AIDS Campaign (an alliance representing over fifty college campuses around the country), veteran ACT UP New York members, people from many different religious communities, activists from Solidarity and Action Against the HIV Infection in India (SAATHII), and more than 500 people, mostly African American, representing ACT UP Philadelphia.[21] The organizing committee that had put the event together was also notably broad, representing AIDS-specific groups including ACT UP, Health GAP, and the Global AIDS Alliance, but also debt relief advocates, such as the Jubilee USA Network, and Africa advocacy groups such as the Washington DC–based lobbying group Africa Action, the oldest group in the United States working on African affairs, and the African Services Committee, a community-based organization located in Harlem founded in 1981 to serve the needs of immigrant and refugee Africans.

The skies opened up on the closing rally, thoroughly drenching the die-hard activists who braved the rain, but even this could not detract from the fact that the June 23 action represented one among a number of high points in a relatively short period of time that seemed to be suggesting that AIDS activist work around the world was seriously paying off. In some ways it resembled the previous year's protest march in Durban, but the lead-up to the march and the meeting that followed it was even more extensive and involved even more international actors within the transnational advocacy network than the Durban meeting had.

This was in part because of the nature of the meeting itself. The purpose of the UN Special Session was to have all the nations in attendance sign a Declaration of Commitment pledging to take specific actions to combat the spread of HIV and provide for those already infected and affected. Predictably, the desirable components of such a declaration look considerably different to different nations and organizations viewing the document. Thus, as with most such documents, the meeting was preceded by months of preparatory negotiations among the countries involved, and AIDS treatment activists in New York City, where the meeting would be held, had been closely monitoring these meetings and negotiations, and disseminating information about their content to their peers throughout the world.

A key feature that has facilitated the creation and maintenance of issue advocacy networks, particularly in the past ten years, has been the rise of the Internet. Although, in a sense, the Internet also highlights and sometimes even deepens the inequality between groups in the global North and South, and between elites and poor activists within developing countries, it is also undeniable that the Internet has been an extraordinarily useful organizing tool. In the case of the UNGASS meeting, not only were preexisting listservs, including Health GAP's, used to facilitate consultation and discussion before, during, and after the UNGASS meeting, but also a listserv run by Health and Development Networks (HDN) was commissioned by UNAIDS to specifically provide a forum, called "Break-the-Silence," for NGO and civil society discussion. These forums also became vehicles for distributing many of the documents put out by Health GAP and other NGOs critical of the content and consultation and negotiation processes of the proposed declaration before the meeting had begun. For example, after examining initial drafts of the declaration, IGLHRC and Health GAP collaborated on a reaction document entitled "Where Are Our Rights?" that focused on the degree to which the declaration seemed to be shying away from explicit statements of the rights of groups infected and at risk from HIV, particularly within marginalized communities. For people unable to be in New York for these collaborations, the ability to scrutinize drafts of the document and of the reaction to it allowed them to have input that would have otherwise been impossible.

As with the Durban AIDS Conference, when treatment activists arrived from around the world, they knew they had entered a target-rich environment. Most of the activists had prepared for the meeting beforehand by applying for either official observer or press status allowing them entry into at least some elements of the Special Session. Two of the clearest targets to emerge were the U.S. government and the international pharmaceutical industry, which had both worked to delete numerous passages within the declaration, including wordings relating to vulnerable populations and the necessity of providing universal AIDS treatment. One symbol of the overlap between these two target groups capitalized upon by activists was the appointment of Henry McKinnell, chairman, CEO, and president of the pharmaceutical giant Pfizer as well as chair of the Pharmaceutical Research and Manufacturers of America, to the official U.S. UNGASS delegation. McKinnell in turn used this position to issue statements opposing the goal of universal treatment access as impractical, arguing, "Trying to put that much money into the system is like pushing on a string. We couldn't spend that money if we had it."[22] The implication that developing countries lacked the "absorptive capacity" for major infusions of resources was particularly galling for many activists from developing countries who had seen, or experienced for themselves, the overcrowded conditions and empty shelves of health care facilities in their home countries

Details of the daily activities of the activists who attended the UNGASS meeting provide a valuable viewing opportunity of the nuts and bolts of how disparate individuals and organizations are able to forge a much more strongly connected transnational network. Essentially, the Special Session worked on some level as a sort of two-tiered conference. At the official level there were three major activities occurring: the fashioning of the Declaration of Commitment that was the stated purpose of the meeting; high-level speeches being made by heads of state, health ministers, and authorities within international governmental organizations; and interactive dialogue sessions in the form of the four Round Tables that had been arranged prior to the opening of the meeting. At the unofficial level, a sort of parallel meeting was occurring in the basement of the United Nations and in adjacent buildings, as accredited observers held and attended presentations, briefing sessions, press conferences, strategy meetings, and other events. The rooms and hallways under and around the United Nations building became the space, literally and figuratively, in which transnational advocacy organizing occurred.

Each day, for example, Health GAP reserved a room in a building across the street from the United Nations for a one-hour strategy meeting with treatment activists around the world about next steps, both at the meeting and beyond, for making treatment a higher priority of governments of the global North and South. This strategy had payoffs not only in the obvious sense of providing opportunities for connecting activists personally and strategically. The official U.S. delegation had a reservation for a daily press conference in the same room for the hour following the treatment access strategy meeting. Naturally, therefore, the treatment activists would stay after their meeting was over, and take front row seats for the daily press conference. It was from this vantage point that they were able to ask (or to call out) questions for the delegation in front of the assembled press. In one particularly memorable exchange, Sheila Kibuka, director of the Kenya-based activist group Hope Africa, took the opportunity to chastise members of the delegation for a statement that had recently been made by USAID Director Andrew Natsios that antiretroviral treatment would be inappropriate for Africans because they lacked a Western view of time. Reminding the delegation of the statement, she prominently identified herself as an African, took off her watch and displayed it, against a backdrop of cheers and applause from her fellow activists in the audience. Such actions were important in the sense that the activists were able to insert alternative interpretations and ideas to the information being given to the press by one of their main targets. But they were also crucial in helping to create the connections between activists who had possibly never met face-to-face before, thereby creating the "density" within the network that Keck and Sikkink note is necessary for it to run optimally.

The UNGASS meeting was called to generally address the HIV/AIDS pandemic; obviously treatment was only one aspect, albeit a very important one, in this larger picture. But the role of Health GAP, which would be expected to focus primarily on the treatment access portion of the meeting, was broadened during the UNGASS meeting for several reasons. One was because of the crucial role that one of its founding members, Karyn Kaplan from the IGLHRC, played at the meeting. Kaplan had been invited to make an official presentation at the Roundtable discussion on Human Rights. But as the meeting drew close, a group of nine countries including Syria, Pakistan, Malaysia, Iran, Libya, and the Vatican registered an official protest and attempted to bar Kaplan from making her presentation specifically because she represented a gay and lesbian group.

Kaplan became a symbol for a larger pattern that many activists had already noted about the meeting and its preparatory events: the exclusion of a number of the very groups whose vulnerability would seem to have suggested that their presence would be imperative at such a global meeting. The grievance list quickly lengthened. It included a wide host of people from developing countries who were detained from attending the meeting, either because their HIV status or their poverty led them to be denied entry visas into the United States. Not only did activists fault the meeting organizers, and the U.S. government particularly, for physically excluding people from the meeting, they also noted that the very mentions of certain critical risk groups were being struck from the Declaration of Commitment being fashioned. Again, mostly at the behest of the same countries that sought to keep Kaplan from speaking at the round table, men who have sex with men (MSM), injection drug users, and sex workers were all being stripped from various versions of the document being debated.

Health GAP became one of the most active groups in fighting against exclusion in several forms. The organization fought on behalf of its own volunteer member, Karyn Kaplan (though she would be speaking in her capacity with IGLHRC). But it also took on the cause of individuals who had being barred from attending because of their HIV status, and of those groups whose very mention was being deleted from the Declaration of Commitment. They did aggressive press work to publicize these exclusions and created a civil society statement protesting the collective exclusionary practices they had experienced, to which approximately ninety organizations—everyone from the World Association of Girl Guides and Girl Scouts to the Manzini Youth of Swaziland to the Sisters of Mercy of the Americas—signed on. They also helped organize a visual protest of the exclusion when, together with several other organizations, including the domestic AIDS advocacy group Housing Works, they produced signs that people could wear to protest the exclusions. A typical sign bore the acronym "MSM" in large letters across most of the paper, and in smaller print at the bottom the words "excluded from the document." The signs were distributed at a morning briefing, and activists wore them throughout their activities for several hours until they were escorted outside by UN security and told they had to remove them in order to regain admittance into the building.

The ultimate results of the antiexclusion activities to which Health GAP and other treatment activists devoted much of their energy were mixed. The would-be NGO observers stopped by the inability to get visas at U.S. embassies remained blocked, just as the references to MSM, sex workers, and injection drug users were never reinserted in the declaration after their removal. On the other hand, Kaplan did address her round-table, following a 62 to 0 vote in the General Assembly, in which many Islamic Countries refused to vote (in an attempt to deny the Assembly a quorum) and some thirty countries abstained. Although some of these activities were tangential to the fight for treatment access, they were essential to the movement-building work that was going on throughout the conference. With each sign-on letter, solidarity protest, and shared experience, the bonds were strengthened between people who mostly had met for the first time a few days ago. The work of getting sign-ons, for example, was also beneficial because it literally facilitated talking among strangers, and after one sign-on was done, a person who had been approached as a stranger the first time could now be spoken to as a colleague to see whether she or he might be interested in being part of a group working on a project or action. Even the overwhelming nature of the work itself could help to forge bonds, as it tended to take place all the time—through meals and coffee breaks and late-night sessions, which allowed people to socialize, albeit in a working context. This became especially important because of a protest that occurred during the meeting on Tuesday June 26 that illustrates the very difficult challenges of doing transnational advocacy work.

Over the course of several strategy sessions a coalition of treatment activist groups determined that they should hold an afternoon press conference to unveil a "treatment manifesto" ending with an element of protest. The conference was scheduled in a conference room within the UN building. A wide variety of groups agreed to endorse and be represented at the press conference, including Oxfam, regional networks such as the Asian Pacific Network of Positive People (APN+), and the Regional Network of People Living with AIDS in Latin America (REDLA), American religious and student groups, ACT UP Paris, and groups from countries including South Africa, Kenya, and Ukraine. The audience was packed with activists who had been given large pill bottles containing pennies and labeled "medications for every nation" which they shook in agreement with the press conference speakers. As the press began to lose interest and leave the press conference, one of the speakers announced that they would be marching to the cafeteria down the hall. The activists walked out of the room chanting loudly and shaking their pill bottles in front of a phalanx of reporters and cameras with a suddenly renewed interest in the event. Members of the UN security staff then headed off much of the group and escorted them out of the building, and once outside, stripped them of their observer credentials. These credentials, in most cases a pass, had been formally applied for, and issued as photo identifications immediately before the conference started. Without them, participants could no longer enter the UN building or take part in any of the satellite or myriad other activities scheduled within the building.

Although the loss of credentials meant that the activists no longer had access to the delegations within the United Nations building, for U.S.-based activists, the demonstration had served an important function. It was well covered by the media and helped to shape the discussion for the remainder of the conference by further raising the salience of treatment. But for activists who had taken part from developing countries, the demonstration carried a much higher level of risk. Many of them had received sponsorship from their country governments, and all of them had been required to apply for visas at the U.S. embassies within their home countries. For them, the loss of their official credentials potentially carried the loss of future opportunities for travel and activist work if the U.S. government or their own country governments chose to be punitive.

U.S.-based treatment activists spent most of the rest of the day working to restore the credentials of their colleagues from developing countries. Although they were successful, Health GAP was criticized online by the International Coordinator of the Global Network of People Living with HIV/AIDS (GNP+), who accused the organization of being "arrogant and disrespectful" in using "People with HIV ... for an agenda." Health GAP issued a conciliatory statement taking responsibility for failing to clearly communicate the potential risks of demonstrating from within the UN, and the ramifications appeared to be short-lived. But they clearly illustrate some of the most problematic issues of working in North-South partnerships, where the costs of punitive action, regardless of the good faith of all the activists involved, falls, as Clifford Bob has suggested, disproportionately heavily on those who are more vulnerable and have fewer resources

STRINGING TOGETHER THE ELEMENTS OF THE TRANSNATIONAL TREATMENT ACCESS MOVEMENT

One very simplified way to think of the transnational treatment access movement that developed in 2000 and 2001 is as a necklace of various-sized beads. The big, and relatively rare, beads were the international events, specifically the 13th International AIDS Conference in Durban and the United Nations Special Session in New York City. Both events were critical from an organizational and substantive perspective. Organizationally, these two conferences afforded treatment activists around the world the opportunity to physically meet, to share skills and successes, and to strategize. Substantively, both international meetings were enormously important for the larger messages that were conveyed by the international media that covered them. In Durban, the "take-away" image was the massive protest of yellow-shirted demonstrators organized by TAC and joined by Western conference attendees demanding treatment. And at the United Nations meeting, the image was that demand seemed to have clearly gained traction, with experts around the globe conceding in public speeches, and the Universal Declaration codifying, that prevention and treatment must go together. The call by UN Secretary General Annan, made before the UN meeting, but widely repeated during it, for a Global Fund to make such treatment financially possible for developing countries further solidified these gains.

Strung together with these two large beads were a host of smaller ones. They represented victorious in-country actions, including South Africa's and particularly TAC's triumph over the branded pharmaceutical companies, as well as Kenya's follow-up victory through legislation, and then Brazil's string of successful showdowns with both individual companies and the U.S. government. Still another "bead" that promised to make even further gains possible was the establishment of the Global Fund for AIDS, Tuberculosis, and Malaria that, by the time of the UN Special Session had already been backed by its future major donors (albeit not at the levels called for by Secretary General Annan).

These country- and project-specific victories were very important for at least three reasons. First, in and of themselves, they are bringing concrete positive benefits, such as drugs and financial support, into the lives of many individuals and societies impacted by HIV/AIDS. Organizationally, they have helped strengthen the ties between elements of the transnational advocacy networks, as organizations and individuals have been able to support one another, often from great distances, as during the Global Day of Action supporting TAC's battle against the pharmaceutical companies in South Africa. And finally, from a chronological perspective, the events have had a cumulative effect, opening up further opportunities within the political structure for later groups to run through (as happened with the Kenya Coalition following on the heels of the TAC victory), and at the same time increasing the cognitive liberation of activists in their beliefs about what is possible.

Importantly, the "string" binding the necklace of events with each other, as well as with other events that predated and would follow these, is a global communication system that makes both coordination of action and daily communication possible in ways unavailable to previous transnational advocacy networks. Web sites for multitudes of organizations maintain vast quantities of information (although much of it is available only in English) and instruction. During some critical moments when an allied set of groups was confronting a hostile government or set of multinational corporations, supporting groups from around the globe (but most commonly in the United States) could go to Web sites that would literally carry "canned protests"—all the materials a group of willing activists would need, from media logos to templates for press releases to step-by-step instructions for carrying off a demonstration. Such easy accessibility of information (easy, at least, for activists in developed countries) has helped to offset the huge advantage held by developed country governments and target corporations, with their vast public relations machines and financial resources available to pay for favorable "spin."

But from the perspective of maintaining a continuous flow of new information and daily contact, nothing has been as critical as listservs. Health GAP maintains a number of listservs, some for internal business, and more for information exchange involving specific campaigns. Many of the organizations with whom Health GAP works closely in the United States, including the Global AIDS Alliance, which maintains a continuing presence in Washington DC and concentrates much of its effort on lobbying there, and the Student Global AIDS Campaign, which coordinates college and high school chapters of student activists around the country, also have their own listservs as well as memberships who participate in both their own organization's list and those of others. The Consumer Project on Technology maintains additional lists about intellectual property issues which are directly relevant to treatment activists, and there are also lists which tend to spring up in preparation for major upcoming international meetings, such as the UN Special Session and the international AIDS conferences. Even more specific are lists that are created to coordinate a particular action or demonstration, such as the J23 list that was explicitly created to aid the planners and participants of the pre–United Nations Special Session march in New York City, and which closed at the conclusion of the event. Still other lists focus on specific regions, such as Africa or Southeast Asia, and others are begun by diaspora communities, such as the Kenya-aids list, which carries postings from Kenya and around the world, but is hosted by a Kenyan living in the United States.

The cross posting among these various lists is extensive, and includes posting of news stories from around the world, strategic and tactical debates, status reports and retrospective analyses, queries, and announcements of meetings and events. Although these lists are the mainstay of the information sharing that Keck and Sikkink note is the lifeblood of transnational advocacy networking, they also serve to reinforce hierarchies within networks and groups. Often it is the ease in accessing computers, and therefore electronically mediated information, that privileges first world activists in the first place, even though their colleagues in developing countries are much more attuned to their own issues and local circumstances. Within groups where there is an unequal distribution of skills and/or money (say with a leader who has higher levels of education and English skills or personal access to the Internet) the same problem can occur

These communication technologies, together with others, particularly cell phones and conference call capabilities, have also been the string holding together Health GAP as an organization. With a highly decentralized structure of a handful of paid staffers living in different cities and supplemented by the labor of approximately twenty extremely active volunteers, it is on regular and frequent conference calls and closed listservs that much strategy and most critical decisions are debated and determined. Together, the phones and computers and technologies that allow people to communicate through them simultaneously have worked to allow the small membership and staff of Health GAP to literally be in many places at once, and to rapidly deploy themselves around the country and the world as campaigns and events have dictated. During all the major international events, and some of the more contained national ones described in this chapter,

representatives of Health GAP were there, helping to organize demonstrations and report conference calls, churning out press releases, orchestrating
behind-the-scenes meetings, and, when all else failed, bending the ears of
decision makers in corridors between these same meetings.

ORGANIZATIONAL STRUCTURE AND DYNAMICS

From mid-2000 through the late summer of 2001 was an exciting time for
Health GAP and for the global treatment access movement. The opportunities created by plummeting ARV prices and increased global financing
opportunities for combating global AIDS were matched with new organizational opportunities within the United States. Other organizations in the
United States were forming, or adding global AIDS to their mission
statements. One such new organization which would share Health GAP's
sense of urgency and willingness to "think big" was the Washington
DC–based organization the Global AIDS Alliance. The group was founded
by physician Paul Zeitz, who had worked for USAID in Zambia and grown
tremendously frustrated with the lack of U.S. urgency about the catastrophe
he saw unfolding within the community he was providing services to. GAA
was established in January 2001, and chose three inaugural projects
including its Global Right to Vital Medicines (MED4ALL) campaign. Like
Health GAP, it has a small staff, but a major commitment to treatment
access, although it also works on several other key issues, including funding
for orphans and vulnerable children.

Arguably even more crucial than the addition of new and important allies
within the movement was Health GAP's own evolution from a loose
coalition to a more formalized (albeit still relatively anarchic) organization.
By mid-2001 Health GAP had been awarded sufficient funding to hire paid
staff. The positions were filled by long-time AIDS activists and ACT UP
veterans Julie Davids, Paul Davis, Asia Russell, and Sharonann Lynch. The
first three were drawn from the ranks of ACT UP Philadelphia and continued to work from that city, while Lynch came from ACT UP New
York. Structurally, Health GAP was established as a project within the
umbrella nonprofit organization Mobilization Against AIDS, based in
San Francisco. But it worked with a high degree of autonomy in its
day-to-day operations, which were directed by a group of "core" volunteer
members, together with the staff, who met through phone conference calls
every two weeks and at weekend-long retreats every four to six months to
make decisions for the organization. Like ACT UP, many individual projects and tasks were taken on by ad hoc working groups within this core,

which would form for the purpose of carrying out a specific campaign or function.

The fact that its entire initial staff, and many of its core volunteers, had their roots (and continue to actively participate) in ACT UP chapters had a major impact on Health GAP, strategically and tactically. On a strategic level, Health GAP has always viewed its role as pushing the boundaries of what might be considered "the possible." As Paul Davis has often noted, "It's the role of Health GAP to be audacious." Initially, this took the form of calling for expanding treatment access to developing countries when it was considered completely impossible, from both affordability and logistical perspectives. Later, when the common wisdom shifted in favor of these claims, it meant aiming for funding numbers others dismissed as ridiculously, unrealistically high, and for pushing for changes at rates others again argued were impossibly fast.

On a personal level, the ACT UP tradition also promoted an internal culture where Health GAP volunteers, and especially staff, pushed themselves to levels that could also be found impossibly ambitious by other groups. Within the group, no one thought it remarkable that even routine conference calls for core and working groups took place in the evenings and on weekends, or that the postings of position papers or proposals would often be dated in the wee hours of the morning, revealing when it was that their authors had finished them. It was equally unremarkable within the group that staff maintained extremely active domestic and international travel schedules, and that they often participated in phone meetings literally as they waited for their flights to be called at various airports.

The organization's breakneck pace, relentless focus on treatment policy outcomes, and ambitious goal-setting has had important implications, good and bad, for Health GAP's interaction with the movement. Admirers have pointed to the organization's capacity to hit the ground running, to achieve important goals quickly, and to provide leadership at the site of political events and conferences, as happened, for example, at the UNGASS meeting. Washington DC–based AIDS advocate Sean Barry once described the Health GAP staff's influence by noting that "people lean in closer when they talk during meetings." In a report commissioned by the Ford Foundation looking at "key players" in the "federal HIV advocacy landscape," Health GAP received high marks for its media presence and overall advocacy effectiveness, but some reservations for its tone and methods. In the report Health GAP is described as having "pursued both an outsider and an insider (less successfully) strategy in the ACT UP mold, with a mix of sophisticated analysis, less sophisticated traditional lobbying and politicking, community protest, and much bravado."[23] But Health GAP's rapid and bold approach has been interpreted as occasionally short-sighted, and even arrogant. For instance, the willingness to take the lead in pushing policy-makers and to take strategic or tactical risks can be resented. The same advocacy report quoted above also noted that Capital Hill staffers singled out Health GAP with complaints: "Their positions are so clear. You can never do enough" and "They're like stone chuckers—they'll throw rocks through my window, then want to come in and meet. They throw around such huge numbers, then bitch and complain, that they lose credibility."[24] Such complaints are arguably predictable from staffers being asked to take political risks, especially ones who do not share Health GAP's philosophies and political orientation.

Criticism from within the advocacy community has also occurred, how-ever, and can be a more serious issue. Health GAP has been accused, sometimes electronically on listservs, and occasionally in face-to-face con-frontations, of not always thinking through the consequences of involving vulnerable developing country activists in risky work. In addition to the story above involving activists being tossed out of the UNGASS meeting, a later corporate campaign targeting Coca-Cola that played out partly in sub-Saharan Africa in which Health GAP was a key organizer would reap similar criticisms. Additionally, and in part because of Health GAP's strategic choice to focus on treatment advocacy, the larger AIDS commun-ity has occasionally voiced concern that Health GAP, and the push for treatment advocacy generally, runs the risk of undermining other parts of the larger AIDS movement by offering a form of "low-hanging fruit" for politicians with antipathy toward many of the movement's more contro-versial goals. Thus, for example, groups particularly concerned about women's reproductive and sexual rights have expressed concern when Health GAP, and a few other treatment groups, have met and worked in shaping legislation with right-wing members of Congress who actively oppose women's reproductive rights and AIDS prevention policies that are not abstinence-based.

The disadvantages of Health GAP's distinctive style were sometimes compounded by inherent features of the inequity between the global North and South. Mistakes were made as Northern and Southern activists tried to find ways to work equally in a global environment where the technological and financial resources gave enormous advantages to the activists from the less-affected countries. The rapid and often reactive nat-ure of campaigns sometimes meant that skill-sharing and leadership devel-opment were sacrificed for the sake of short-term victories. Additionally, the strong leadership of some of the global treatment activists was both a strength and a weakness. On the one hand, it meant that there were courageous, articulate figures willing to publicly take on much more powerful and better financed opponents. But it also often meant that there were personality conflicts within the movement among these leaders, who sometimes had differing views of tactics and strategy, and who often did not have the luxury of extensive face time to resolve differences. The Internet is an excellent, rapid conduit for information, but it is less useful as a conveyer of nuance and tone, which are easily lost or misinterpreted in the process. Despite these challenges, by late summer 2001, the transnational advocacy network had clearly been strengthened by the events of the preceding year, and was moving into the fall with strong momentum. But then on September 11, a small group of terrorists would hijack four American planes and, in a single morning, wreak an abrupt and seismic shift on the politics of the United States and, ultimately, the world.

Chapter 4

Win Some, Keep Going: Sustaining Global AIDS Treatment Activism

I n the days that followed the September 11 attack, the shock and sadness of the nation was soon accompanied by a new fear of what might come next. By early October 2001, the ruins of the World Trade Center were still smoldering and repairs had barely begun on the side of the Pentagon that terrorists had demolished. Although definitive counts of the death toll had not yet been reached, attention was already turned to the number and form of possible future casualties in the widely expected follow-up assaults. Televised talking heads and ordinary citizens in coffee shops speculated widely about the most likely next target. Would it be a plane crash into a nuclear power plant? A radiological "dirty bomb" in Times Square, at Disneyworld, or during the World Series? Maybe even a crude nuclear device smuggled in through an unchecked shipping container, exploding on the docks of Los Angeles, New York, Seattle, or New Orleans?

But when the next terrorist attacks did come, they did so silently, through means as mundane as the daily mail delivery. "On October 2, 2001, a 63-year old Caucasian photo editor working for a Florida newspaper awoke early with nausea, vomiting, and confusion and was taken to a local emergency room for evaluation. . . . The patient died on October 5. Autopsy findings . . . showed disseminated *Bacillus anthracis* in multiple organs." The case was puzzling because there had not been a case of infection with *B. anthracis*—more commonly know as anthrax—in the United States since 1976. Although it had been a scourge of the wool and tanning industries in the eighteenth and nineteenth centuries, when humans inhaled or touched anthrax spores when in contact with sheep, inhalational anthrax had been diagnosed only eighteen times in all of the twentieth century in the United States.[1]

The case might have been written off as a fluke if public health authorities had not learned that a 73-year-old mailroom clerk who had delivered mail to the deceased photo editor had also been hospitalized in late September. And then in mid-October, a series of U.S. Postal Service employees in Washington DC and New Jersey all began to experience flu-like symptoms that rapidly worsened, leading to death in several. By that time, suspicious letters containing white powder had begun to appear in the offices of powerful figures in media, including the editor of the *New York Post* and the offices of NBC News anchor Tom Brokaw. And then on October 15, 2001, an intern opened a letter laced with anthrax in the Hart Senate Office building of Tom Daschle, the Senate Majority Leader.[2]

After some initial confusion, the offices of the members of both the House and the Senate were closed and sealed off immediately, and medical teams in protective clothing and respirators were sent in to search for evidence of anthrax. Twenty-eight Senate staffers would eventually test positive for exposure to levels of infection up to 3,000 times the known lethal dose of anthrax. All of them survived—as did thousands of potentially exposed postal workers and other government workers—after immediately being put on a regimen of ciprofloxin, or Cipro as it is more commonly called, which was the most effective known treatment, although it was believed that other antibiotics might also be effective. The Hart Building would remain closed for three months, and the Environmental Protection Agency would eventually estimate clean-up costs at $41.7 million. Above all, the ability of Congress to fully function was crippled at a time of national crisis.[3]

The anthrax outbreak would have constituted a genuine public health emergency under any circumstances. Against the backdrop of the September 11 attacks it was inevitably seen as a second—and probably not the last—wave of a sustained assault on the United States, this time by means as different as possible from the violence of airplanes being crashed into buildings. Laboratory tests soon determined that the anthrax spores in the letters had been highly refined, some said "weaponized," so that they could waft freely through the air and infect people more efficiently. Some particles were so small that they could even escape a sealed envelope, explaining the infections found among postal workers, and no one knew how many more contaminated letters had already been mailed or were on their way. With mail being carried to virtually every building in the country, it seemed that terrorists had found a way to reach every corner of the United States.

Finding supplies of Cipro to treat a limited number of cases proved manageable with existing stocks of the medication, but what if the number of people appearing in hospital emergency rooms increased drastically? Although the low-tech delivery of anthrax via the mail had thus far suggested a greater desire to cause panic than death, caution dictated the need to have massive supplies of Cipro at the ready—enough to treat 10 million people, estimated U.S. Secretary of Health and Human Services Tommy Thompson. With a full course of 120 days of medication, this would amount to 1.2 billion pills of Cipro. But the production capacity of the patent holder, pharmaceutical giant Bayer, was only 2 million pills per day, meaning that it would take 600 days to produce 1.2 billion pills.[4]

Senator Charles Schumer of New York was the first major U.S. political figure to find it unacceptable for the United States to wait up to two years for Bayer to produce adequate supplies of Cipro. On October 16, he called for the United States to invoke its statutory authority to issue a compulsory license in the face of a public health emergency and allow three or more other manufacturers to begin producing generic versions of the drug even as Bayer maintained its exclusive patent for commercial sales of Cipro. "We cannot just rely on Bayer to ensure we have a sufficient supply of Cipro," said Schumer in a statement, noting that it was dangerous to rely on a single manufacturer and that generic versions would be much less expensive.[5] Three days later, the Canadian government did just what Schumer had called for: overrode Bayer's patent and ordered a million generic-version pills from a Canadian supplier. "These are extraordinary and unusual times. Canadians expect and demand that their government will take all steps necessary to protect their health and safety," said a spokesperson for Health Canada.[6]

The storm passed almost as quickly as it arose. No more anthrax attacks occurred after that date, the need for massive stockpiles of Cipro never materialized, and as of this writing, the entire case remains unsolved. Faced with the threat that their patent might be broken, Bayer quickly dropped the price per pill from the usual government price of $1.77 to $0.95 for the first 100 million tablets, with further price cuts down to $0.85 and $0.75 for subsequent orders. In the end, fewer than a dozen Americans contracted anthrax, of whom five died—roughly the same number of Africans who died from AIDS every minute. Yet the point had been made clearly: when the public health emergency occurs in the United States, all bets are off. Although the U.S. government never ended up breaking the patent on Cipro, it successfully pressured Bayer for a major price decrease and kept open the door for breaking the patent should a widescale crisis actually come to pass.

By coincidence, the anthrax scare occurred less than a month before another major meeting of the WTO, this one scheduled for Doha, the capital city of the Middle Eastern country of Qatar and a location that could much more easily be shielded from the massive protests that had marked other WTO meetings. And also largely by coincidence, a top priority of developing nations and AIDS activists at the Doha meeting was the clarification of Article 31 of the TRIPS agreement, which allows the breaking of patents in "situations of national emergency or other circumstances of extreme urgency." The timing was fortuitous, because the United States could hardly have experienced the urgency of the issue more clearly. Nor could the activists have asked for a better example to point out the hypocrisy of the United States in moving almost immediately toward breaking patents for a *hypothetical* health crisis while fighting relentlessly to keep much poorer countries from breaking patents for a raging actual health crisis.

MAINTAINING THE MOMENTUM

The treatment activists churning out press releases on the hypocritical stance of the United States at the same time they were buying their plane tickets destined for Doha knew they were operating in a political landscape that had changed dramatically over a short period of time in two ways. Most immediately, September 11 significantly altered the political opportunity structure for not only the treatment access movement but for all protest movements in the United States. The near-total fixation of the American media on terrorism in general, and the September 11 attacks in particular, virtually overnight rendered competing stories minor at best, invisible at worst. Additionally, many of the tried and true tactics of the activist's "toolbag"—from mass protest to open criticism of government policy to (and especially) civil disobedience—were viewed in the new political atmosphere as unpatriotic and morally suspect. In some cases, they also carried more risk, as national, state, and municipal authorities passed new legislation, or enforced old regulations with new vigor.

Despite these setbacks, there was another political reality that was also important. The global treatment access movement has always focused on fostering two key developments in order to universalize access to AIDS medications. The first such development was the meteoric drop of prices of these drugs, and the second was the conversion of donors to be willing to pay for these newly discounted products. By fall 2001 the global treatment access movement had proof that both conditions could happen, and indeed, on at least a limited scale, were already in place. The phenomenal success of Brazil in making its own generic medications and providing them free of charge to its citizens, together with the Indian company Cipla's February 2001 announcement of even lower prices than Brazil's, was widely trumpeted by activists, and repeated in the mainstream press and among global policymakers. A drop in price from the $10,000-plus annual pricetag widely cited for triple therapy in the United States to $350 is clearly a change of immense proportions; as a news event it set the stage for making a vastly expanded treatment vision seem much more attainable.

The initiation of the Global Fund (together with the previous decision by the World Bank to change its policies to allow its loans to go for the purchase of generic drugs) provided a critical mechanism to make the vision happen. The Global Fund's operations began with its first board meeting in January 2002, and its first set of grants was announced in April. Although it was called for by UN Secretary General Annan, it is actually not a part of the UN. Rather it is run by a board drawn from donor and recipient country governments, foundations, the private sector, and NGOs. It exists to raise money from donors, mainly but not exclusively developed countries, and disperse the money to countries seeking to prevent and treat AIDS, tuberculosis, and malaria among their citizens. A unique feature of the Global Fund is the process it has created for making grants. Grants are based on proposals not from country governments but rather from Country Coordinating Mechanisms. These bodies are expected to be composed of key stakeholders within the country—including representatives from government (especially ministries of health), but also NGOs, the private sector, and, critically, people living with the three diseases. (In extreme cases, NGOs may bypass this mechanism to make a proposal directly, but this is rare.) These proposals are first reviewed by an independent Technical Review Panel, composed of international health experts, and favorably reviewed proposal are then forwarded to the board for final decisions.[7]

Having realized huge price cuts *and* funding mechanisms, what the movement needed to do next was expand and institutionalize these critical gains. In practical terms this meant two things: removing as many barriers to the use of generic medications as possible and at the same time ramping up efforts to get money for these drugs—whether from multilateral sources like the Global Fund, unilateral donations from countries, corporations, and charities, or poor countries, own resources (freed up by canceling external debts). It was with these aims firmly in mind that activists geared up for the next confrontation, to be played out in the tightly secured conference halls of Doha, Qatar.

PUBLIC CONCESSIONS AND PRIVATE REVERSALS AT DOHA

In many respects, the WTO meeting that convened in Doha on November 9 was radically different from the previous one in Seattle. Most notably, the masses of protesters from a broad coalition of antiglobalization forces that had propelled the Seattle meeting into history were now visually represented by a tiny contingent consisting of only the Greenpeace ship *Rainbow Warrior* and a small handful of activists outside the conference center. Activist NGOs which were accredited to officially attend were severely limited to one representative per organization—reportedly because of lack of accommodation.[8] Additionally, the mood that had characterized the meeting a year ago, marked by exuberant and broad criticism of the multinational corporations and the American government, considered by protesters to be their chief representative, was gone. In its place was a palpable fear among many of being seen to be in alliance with the terrorists through open criticism of the government of the country they attacked. A September 27 *New York Times* article had noted that a wide variety of activist and advocacy organization had started pulling their punches, canceling actions, and muting statements that might be perceived as critical and therefore, unpatriotic.

In AIDS politics, these fears had already compelled the international NGO Oxfam to pull an online petition targeting the United States in the run-up to the Doha meeting. The petition had been designed before September 11, and had singled out the United States for its strong stance in favor of patented medicines. Featuring a prominent "Uncle Sam" graphic, it had been developed together with Health GAP and the TRIPS Action Network, and it called on the United States to "put health before wealth." Although the petition was reinstituted a week later, it had been substantially reworked, replacing the cartoon of Uncle Sam with a pill bottle picture, and taking out the wording that had situated the United States in the spotlight for criticism. The fear of being negatively perceived was accompanied by an additional fear—that of not being noticed at all. Health GAP staffer Asia Russell's frustration was evident in her remarks to the press when she said, "What we find is a blackout on coverage and attention to activism."[9]

It was in this difficult environment that treatment activists converged on the meeting hall in Doha. Absent the throngs of protesters making demands and using splashy statements and actions to garner media attention, and in the constrained media atmosphere of the time, activists emphasized a different set of strategies, centered heavily on continuous interactions, begun before the WTO meeting, with developing country delegations. This tactic was not appreciated by developed country delegations, who complained that the NGOs were encouraging "unrealistic" negotiating positions by getting developing countries "wound up."[10] Nor did they enjoy the relentless face-to-face pressure on negotiators from the United States and Europe, who were literally buttonholed and surrounded at various times and who reluctantly gave in to sit-down meetings with activist groups as a result. In an ironic twist on the Keck and Sikkink "boomerang" model discussed previously, activists from the global North were able to use a developing country government to pressure their own more intransigent governments. Their critical ally was the team representing the government of Brazil, which also sent high-level health and AIDS officials to the meeting.

Despite the initially unpromising setting of the meeting, activists had worked mightily beforehand to align the stars in their favor, and it paid off. In addition to the crucial alliance between activist coalitions and the Brazilian government, there was the rhetorical argument created by the U.S. government's hypocritical stance on Cipro, which Brazilian AIDS Program Head Paulo Teixeira recalled bringing up repeatedly. And the decision of eighty developing country governments to stand together, egged on by activists, allowed them to push for the ability to override patent rights in manufacturing drugs not only for AIDS, but also for other illnesses.[11]

Although the pharmaceutical industry sent specific instructions in the form of a letter from industry lobby head Alan Holmer to U.S. Trade Representative Robert Zoellick against compromises affecting the strength of patents, the Doha round would go down as a victory, though not a complete one, in the activist/developing country column. The source of this win was found in Paragraph 4 of the document which was adopted at the conference, entitled as the "Declaration on the TRIPS Agreement and Public Health," and subsequently referred to by activists as the "Doha Declaration." It specifically elevates the cause of public health, stating "that the TRIPS agreement does not and should not prevent members from taking measures to protect public health" and that "the Agreement can and should be interpreted and implemented in a manner supportive of WTO Members' right to protect public health, and in particular, to support access to medicines for all."[12]

Reactions by the victors ranged from unqualified enthusiasm to cautious optimism. Consumer Project on Technology Director Jamie Love jubilantly likened it to a transcription of demonstrator signs straight into the Doha Declaration. In a more cautious assessment to the public listserv maintained by Health GAP, staffer Asia Russell voiced reservations, noting that the United States, Switzerland, the European Union, and Japan had all managed to water down language within the document. Even more seriously, PhRMA had succeeded, via the U.S. delegation, to push off for another meeting the critical question of compulsory license for export, which would allow generic drug producing countries to export their products to poor countries without the capabilities of producing their own generics.

This final caveat would prove to be critical. Much of what the U.S. government and the pharmaceutical industry "gave away" in the headlines covering the Doha Declaration they managed to quietly recoup at later meetings and, more important, in bilateral trade agreements with a whole raft of countries and regions in the following two years. These subsequent agreements have enlisted a host of additional conditions that make it more difficult for the countries signing the bilateral agreements to actually avail themselves of the gains of the Doha agreements. Among the conditions placed on these bilateral deals are limitations to compulsory licensing, increasing what is considered "patentable," extending the terms of patents beyond what the WTO requires, and eliminating the right to parallel import (which is essential for countries that do not have the internal capacity to manufacture drugs themselves).

The dynamics of these later developments after the victory at Doha illustrate the strengths and weaknesses of transnational advocacy networks generally, and of the global treatment access movement in particular. Transnational advocacy places a heavy emphasis on information and symbolic politics, where the ability to frame an issue in a simple, emotionally and morally compelling way is what helps compensate for the enormous inequity of resources between activists and their targets. In the run-up to the Doha meeting, activists were able to play on several tactical advantages—the centrality of the meeting and of the common stakes of many developing countries, and the relative simplicity and moral clarity of the message: health of the poor before the profits of rich corporations. The trade strategy to move to bilateral and regional trade agreements, and to negotiate more technical provisions, effectively negates both these advantages. It is harder to rally a critical mass of global activists around a country-specific case (and this is further complicated by the multiple nature of these cases, which dissipates a limited pool of activist expertise and resources). It is also harder to frame the language and substance of technical negotiations in simple, morally compelling terms that appeal to other activists and especially to broader publics.

FACING OFF IN BARCELONA

Following the landmark International AIDS Conference in Durban, South Africa, in 2000, the conference returned to the global north, and was hosted in July 2002 in Barcelona, Spain. As with previous conferences, thousands of scientists, clinicians, and other experts would attend and hold panels, poster sessions, round tables, and discussions. But for the treatment activist community, Barcelona would be remembered primarily for two reasons: first, for the international opening of a new kind of corporate campaign in the struggle for access to medicines and, second, for a protest inside the conference hall that would lay bare the level of animosity between the Bush administration and the majority of the AIDS advocacy community.

The decision to explicitly target a giant multinational corporation was in one sense nothing new. In fact, protesting the pharmaceutical corporation Burroughs Wellcome (now, several mergers later, the even larger GlaxoSmithKline) had been the inaugural action of the fledging ACT UP New York chapter that founded the movement. But up until 2002 AIDS treatment activists had largely limited the scope of their anticorporate activities to the pharmaceutical industry. This limit had been intentional, and was based on several considerations. One strictly pragmatic consideration had been the question of limited resources. Given the paucity of volunteers, and especially paid staff (recall that for most of its history Health GAP has operated with only three full-time staffers), organizations within the treatment access movement have had to triage their campaigns and targets. And, especially after the Seattle WTO meeting, there were clearly other organizations and activists willing to take on multinational corporations in a variety of ways. In addition to these practical considerations, there were ideological concerns. Health GAP and other treatment access groups operate mainly from a rights-based perspective that considers health care, including access to effective medicines, a basic human right. As with other human rights, the primary responsibility for their provision resides with government, and so governments, from both developed and developing countries, are pressured to provide for the world's citizenry.

By 2002, however, treatment activists began to examine the case for targeting multinational companies beyond the pharmaceutical industry. On a practical level, the fact that allies and potential allies were already leveling demands at corporations could be looked at in a new way. Rather than viewing it as an area that was "already covered," the nonpharmaceutical corporate sector could potentially be highly vulnerable to negative publicity regarding AIDS policies.

Another reason that a corporate target seemed more attractive is that a new group of activists had emerged to help provide the energy and bodies for a campaign. By this point, a nascent student movement around global AIDS had developed. It began in Boston as the convergence of several AIDS-related activist efforts, with the Boston Global Action Network's Africa AIDS Project coming out of the larger organization's antiglobalization work. Among the key figures of the Africa AIDS Project was Northeastern University law professor Brook Baker, who later became a leading volunteer within Health GAP. At Harvard University, two mobilizations were underway as students were simultaneously organizing as both undergraduates and within the Kennedy School, the latter under the leadership of graduate student Adam Taylor. These three organizational efforts came together collectively for a brief period, most notably for a protest at the offices of the pharmaceutical company Pfizer on World AIDS Day (December 1) 2000.

However, the student-led part of the movement moved away from the antiglobalization path in which BGAN was rooted and incorporated as a nonprofit organization known as Global Justice. Global Justice's first campaign was the Student Global AIDS Campaign (SGAC), which was quickly expanded to other campus chapters and a national office in Washington with the help of a grant from the Bill and Melinda Gates Foundation. Although SGAC had a decidedly less activist orientation than Health GAP or ACT UP (which was a reason for its split from BGAN in the first place), it did have contacts with interested students from a nationwide network of college campuses. A campaign against a prominent multinational corporation was viewed as a potential bridge to bring students together with the more experienced activists of the treatment access movement. Such a campaign could be presented to college students as a logical follow-up to the successful antiapartheid divestment campaigns on college campuses in the 1980s. Additionally, colleges themselves could be a key factor in a campaign targeting Coca-Cola because of its intense competition with rival Pepsi for exclusive marketing rights on individual college campuses. A "Kick Coke Off Campus" Campaign might make Coke marketing executives worry in a way that a less targeted call for a boycott would not.

In addition to the shift in tactical considerations afforded by new potential allies, there were new ideological considerations to consider. A number of the global corporations most heavily impacted by AIDS can also be implicated as strongly influencing its spread for a variety of reasons ranging from practices that disrupt the social fabric of communities and families to conducting operations (such as trucking) that physically facilitate the spread of the virus. A classic example is the mining companies of South Africa, whose employment policies, such as offering only the barest of housing to its direct employees and none to families who are often situated far from the mines, actually *create* the conditions that foster the spread of HIV. Thus, a campaign against a well-selected multinational corporation could also be used to expose culpability and demand accountability for the exploitative practices of corporations.

In June 2001 Coca-Cola publicly announced that it would "partner" with UNAIDS in using its resources to combat AIDS in Africa. Although the announcement was accompanied by a flurry of corporate press releases and consequent flattering stories in *The Wall Street Journal* and *New York*

Times, it also became the opportunity that activists considering starting a corporate campaign had been looking for.[13] At issue was a semantic sleight of hand that activists quickly pounced upon: although Coke had long taken credit for its status as one of the largest employers in sub-Saharan Africa, this claim rested on the counting of employees of its bottlers throughout the region as members of the Coke "family." Yet in the much-touted treatment announcements, these employees found themselves entirely excluded. Coke intended to offer treatment only to its 1,200 "direct" employees, leaving out the 60,000–100,000 (estimates varied according to who was counting) employees of the bottlers. The considerations had already been piling up: Coke had huge name recognition; it was vulnerable in precisely the area from which new activists could be recruited (i.e., college campuses); a change in policy to extend treatment could positively affect thousands of lives and impact the practices of other major employers. But it was Coke's own duplicitous representation of what it was doing that sealed the decision. In the debate over whether to focus on a corporation such as a mining or oil company whose practices could more explicitly be linked to complicity in spreading HIV/AIDS or a giant with huge name recognition, Coca-Cola's headline-grabbing actions gave the company the edge on this particular dubious distinction.

And so, activists launched an offensive against Coke's grandstanding at Coca-Cola's annual shareholder's meeting in April 2002. But the campaign kicked into high gear in June with a colorful confrontation that was, in the words of a joint ACT UP–Health GAP press release, "by land and by sea." The setting was a showy gala on Pier 60 in New York City, with corporate representatives being feted at an awards ceremony sponsored by the Global Business Council, with a guest list that included Kofi Annan, Bill Clinton, and emcee Dan Rather. Inside the event, activists managed to interrupt the ceremony and loudly challenge the "exemplary" nature of these award-winning policies; in the words of Eric Sawyer, "Multinational corporations have no laurels to rest on. . . . Medical apartheid is nothing to be proud of." This "medical apartheid" label, a slogan meant to cast shame on the global double standard of treatment for the rich and excuses of "too expensive" for the rest, would become an important way of representing the impact of Coke's announced policy that would give treatment to white, upper-class office workers but not to African working-class bottlers and truckers. At the same time that activists were disrupting the ceremony inside, their colleagues floated alongside the pier using bullhorns to chant "Coke lies, workers die, AIDS treatment now!"

The Barcelona meeting offered a perfect opportunity to globalize the campaign. Health GAP and ACT UP activists headed to Barcelona loaded down with not only the usual black T-shirts and laptop computers but also an unwieldy new prop—a twenty-five foot Coca-Cola helium balloon emblazoned with signs accusing Coke of medical apartheid. Although activists maintained the balloon and distributed information throughout the week, on July 10 they held a protest, carrying signs and chanting as they proceeded through the exhibition hall and ended with a spirited rally. The rally was also used as the opportunity to formally announce the formation of a global coalition of activists, including groups from the United States (Health GAP, ACT UP New York and Philadelphia, and the Global AIDS Alliance), South Africa (Treatment Action Campaign), France (ACT UP Paris), Morocco (Association Morocaine de Lette Contre le SIDA), and Thailand (Thai Network of People Living with HIV), as well as the European AIDS Treatment Group with representatives from thirty-one nations. This new coalition proclaimed its plan to hold a global day of action to protest Coke's HIV/AIDS workplace policies in developing countries.

Of course, the fact that Health GAP and other treatment activists had decided to open a corporate campaign by taking on Coca-Cola did not mean that they were abandoning any of their more traditional targets. As numerous papers and AIDS community reporting services chronicled, International AIDS Conferences have become predictable sites for protests of all sizes, and Barcelona was no exception. ACT UP chapters from both the United States and Paris often had a leading role in organizing and executing these actions. An Agence France Presse (AFP) wire story, "Protests Mark AIDS Conference for Third Day Running," typifies the coverage, noting protests against not only Coca-Cola, but also the Catalonian government, the European Commission, pharmaceutical company GlaxoSmithKline and the Health Minister of France and U.S. Secretary of Health and Human Services (HHS).[14]

Of all these actions, it was the one aimed at HHS Secretary Tommy Thompson that marked the conference most indelibly. Fully twelve years had passed since a U.S. president had sent a high-level representative to an International AIDS Conference. Back in 1990 the first President Bush sent HHS Secretary Louis Sullivan to San Francisco, where he was roundly booed by the audience during his attempt to deliver a speech. Now sitting in the first row in Barcelona, he watched his successor face a similar, though even more extreme, fate. The protest began as Thompson came to the podium. This was the cue for activists in the audience to begin blowing whistles and hurling cries of "Shame, shame" and "No more lies" at the stage. There were a number of demands, reflected in the chants led by the protesters: "Where's the ten billion?" (a reference to the actual estimated needs of the Global Fund), "Clean needles now," and "Money for AIDS, not for war." As Thompson continued to attempt to deliver his thirty minute address that no one could hear, approximately thirty activists came up on the stage with signs protesting Bush and Thompson's "Murder and neglect" and demanding more money for the Global Fund to Fight AIDS, Tuberculosis, and Malaria.

What was most remarkable about this event, however, was not the actions of the original protests. It was the audience reaction. Although there were some members of the audience who clearly disapproved of the interruptions (including former Secretary Sullivan, who sat stone-faced through the disruption and later denounced the action as "mindless advocacy"), the protesters unleashed a wave of pent-up anger in the audience aimed at the administration. T. Richard Corcoran, a Health GAP volunteer, recalled the surprisingly high support from the audience. He and a handful of other volunteers had been outside the auditorium, working at a furious pace to get out copies of a flier signed by twelve organizations, together with additional information in press kits to explain why the protestors were interrupting the speech. Yet these very explanations had been supplanted by the enthusiastic joining in of the audience with "all these people who don't usually do this sort of thing standing up and pointing at the stage shouting 'shame, shame' at the top of their lungs."[15] At the conclusion of the protest, when the activists left the stage, the audience clapped in support. Interestingly, there was no attempt by anyone to stop the protestors when they came on stage with their signs, no public reference to the protests in the speeches of either Richard Feachem (Director of the Global Fund) or Gro Harlem Brundtland (Director of the World Health Organization), who followed Thompson on the stage, and no public criticism during the remainder of the day.[16]

If the reaction in Spain was muted, however, the same could not be said for the response within some circles of the U.S. government, within both the Congress and the executive branch. Thompson was reportedly livid, and considered the activists particularly ungrateful in light of the recent initiative of the Bush administration to spend 500 million dollars on reducing mother-to-child transmission in Africa and the Caribbean. During the remainder of the summer following the conference, twelve members of Congress directed the Department of Health and Human Services to review the federal funding of both the International AIDS Conference and of government and nongovernmental groups from the United States who attended. This letter was followed by a request from a staffer of a House Government Reform Subcommittee specifically questioning federal funding levels of sixteen AIDS community groups, including the twelve that signed the flier explaining the reason for the Thompson protest.

The angry reaction within government, however, had multiple interpretations. Those sympathetic to the administration couched their complaints as objections to Thompson's free speech rights being abridged, and
the "misuse" of government funds to finance groups that publicly dissented
from government policy. Yet activists saw something different: behind the
anger lurked the unmistakable fact that the activists had clearly gotten the
attention of the administration. Rather than pulling their punches, they
pushed on. Having publicly called out the administration as shamefully
derelict in its global AIDS obligations, activists now decided to work to
shape the alternative reality they sought.

The form of the new advocacy vehicle was a proposal originated by
activists but dubbed the Presidential AIDS Initiative. The initiative was
drafted with three components: access to affordable medicines; prevention
services and support for affected communities (including mother-to-child
prevention and the empowerment of women and girl children); and adequate financial resources (including a $2.5 billion budget request for FY04
for global AIDS, with half for the Global Fund, and debt cancellation for
heavily AIDS-impacted impoverished nations). The proposal rapidly gained
widespread support from over 300 endorsing local, national, and international organizations. In late November as an early observance of
World AIDS Day, activists also organized a protest bringing hundreds of
marchers to protest in front of the White House. The protestors delivered
mock body bags, while a group of thirty-one individuals, including
the executive directors of Africa Action and Housing Works, as well as
the entire staff of Health GAP, chained themselves together and conducted
a die-in for which they were arrested.

COCA-COLA: THE STRUGGLE CONTINUES

Meanwhile, as the work on the Presidential AIDS Initiative unfolded, the
campaign against Coca-Cola was also in full swing, with organizing efforts
and outreach to possible allies, particularly student groups, underway. On
July 22, ACT UP Atlanta, which had, like many other chapters, fallen silent
in the late 1990s, was reactivated with a spirited protest at Coca-Cola's
world headquarters. Working in partnership with southern students
belonging to the Student Global AIDS Campaign, as well as several pro-
labor groups protesting Coke's union policies in South America, they drew
a crowd of approximately one hundred people in front of the office
headquarters. Before the gathering and two hour performance complete
with performance artists and a "Choke-a-Cola" mascot, activists had also
managed to unfurl a fifty foot banner from the Fifth Street bridge reading

"Coke adds death: AIDS drugs for Coke workers now!" Although Sonya Soutus, Coca-Cola's director of corporate communications, dismissed the charges as "relatively misleading" since the employees in question were "not Coca-Cola's direct employees," ACT UP Atlanta members referred to the event as "just the beginning."[17]

On September 26, Coca-Cola changed tack and announced a new plan that would split the costs of covering employee and spouse health care benefits, including antiretrovirals, with the local bottlers. Although Coke campaigners hailed the announcement as a positive development, they noted that the plan as announced did not yet include all the bottlers, that it did not cover the children of employees, and that the copayment that was expected of covered employees would be a serious hardship in areas where wages are very low.[18] Significantly, they decided to forge ahead with the Global Day of Action to which they had publicly committed themselves, scheduled to be held on October 17.

In preparation for the big day, AIDS activists from Health GAP, ACT UP, SGAC, the Global AIDS Alliance and others had availed themselves of a full palate of the options available to modern transnational movements. For months, beginning after the Barcelona meeting, a working group of U.S. campaigners had been phone conferencing on at least a twice-monthly basis to strategize, make decisions in the face of emerging events, and coordinate logistical work. Day-to-day communication took place on a listserv entirely devoted to AIDS activism targeting multinational corporations, and cell phones (and less, frequently, the Internet) made it possible to keep global campaigners from developing countries connected as well. Plans for the day were equally varied and tied to the groups organized in the United States and around the world. Students at twelve college campuses in the United States and Canada announced plans to participate in ways as disparate as "guerilla flyering" of on-campus Coke machines at Iowa State to more sedate presentations of petitions to university presidents, chancellors, and student governments at a host of schools. In California, the District of Columbia, Georgia, Massachusetts, Pennsylvania, New York, Vermont, and Washington, students either joined protests with fellow activists in major cities or held their own on campuses. There were larger community-based protests around the country as well. In Atlanta protesters converged in front of the World of Coke Museum with banners and "Medical Apartheid" Coke machines. In New York City the twenty-five-foot Barcelona Coke balloon was resurrected by 400 activists, this time in partnership with a mock figure of CEO Douglas Daft heaving thirty-two body bags (one for each African bottling plant not providing treatment) at Coca-Cola's Manhattan office. In San Francisco, ACT UP

East Bay and Health GAP organized a protest rally in front of the Pacific Stock Exchange, and in Washington DC Health GAP, the Global AIDS Alliance, and the Student Global AIDS Campaign joined forces to put together a protest featuring a giant coffin and moving graveyard.

Across the ocean, activists in other parts of the world were ensuring that the seventeenth would be remembered as a truly global event. In France, members of ACT UP Paris managed to shut down the Coke factory in Grigny. After climbing fences and hanging banners, they succeeded in blocking workers from entering and created a vivid visual display from a large map of Africa which they covered in Coke cans and fake blood. The Japan-Africa Forum launched a petition drive and delivered a memorandum to Coke representatives in Tokyo. And in the epicenter of the controversy, Africa itself, a number of activist groups in Burkina Faso, Mali, Morocco, and Togo took action as well. Some conducted rallies while others, judging the situation to be too dangerous, conducting press work and low-key lobbying with Coke and Ministry of Health officials.

The overall success of the day, in terms of coordination, media coverage, and general good feeling of solidarity among new and old activists was marred by one frightening situation that occurred the day before and served as a cruel reminder of the inequality between activists and their targets. In Ghana, a peaceful protest had been planned, and the Ghana AIDS Treatment Access Group (GATAG) had petitioned the police for a permit two weeks in advance of the protest. On the day before the scheduled protest, activists from GATAG had a conversation with Coca-Cola representatives, who claimed that they were being misinformed by Health GAP. Later the same day a leader of GATAG was arrested and brought to police headquarters for interrogation. This information was conveyed by e-mail from an African activist to Sharonann Lynch, the Health GAP staffer leading up the Coke Campaign. What followed was an intensive afternoon of back-and-forth communication, phone and e-mail communication, between Lynch, the activist, the Global Business Council and UNAIDS (both of which had been called by Lynch to intercede), and Robert Lindsay, the Ghanaian Vice President for Coca-Cola Africa. Although Lindsay continuously denied any involvement in the arrest and the accompanied threats by police against the activists, other global activists from around the world responded to listserv requests to call both the Ghanaian police and Coca-Cola Ghana to demand the release of the Ghanaian NGO leader. They also made less diplomatically worded calls to Coca-Cola's Atlanta headquarters to complain against the intimidation of the Ghanaian protesters. By the end of the day, to the relief of his fellow global colleagues, news came of the activist's release. Although the programs would not roll out as fast, or as comprehensively, as treatment activists would have liked, eventually many of the bottlers did create treatment programs. But the October Global Day of Action incident served as a stark reminder to all of the very real dangers that activists faced, particularly in the global South, in pressing for treatment.

NEW SURPRISES

As both the Coke Campaign and the push for a Presidential AIDS Initiative clearly illustrate, the model inherited from ACT UP and other AIDS advocacy groups still worked well in pursuing global goals. Health GAP and other groups pushed the envelope with protest and civil disobedience, while at the same time broadening grassroots support through lower-cost vehicles such as organizational sign-ons and endorsements and conducting traditional lobbying work and production of white papers and products for the media. Within the movement, some division of labor was happening. The Global AIDS Alliance, for instance, an organization slightly younger than Health GAP, but based in Washington DC was active in much of the day-to-day lobbying that needed to occur on Capitol Hill. Several large AIDS service organizations, such as New York City's Gay Men's Health Crisis, and international nongovernmental organizations such as MSF/Doctors Without Borders were involved in forging strategy, and trade expert groups, especially the Consumer Project on Technology and Essential Action, offered technical expertise. Groups that had been less AIDS-focused in the 1990s now also emerged to help with the enormous workload, including RESULTS (an advocacy organization seeking to end hunger and the worst effects of poverty) and the Center for Health and Gender Equity (CHANGE).

The work continued to be coordinated primarily through conference calls, including a twice-monthly strategy call hosted by Health GAP, and e-mail listservs. Additionally, in Washington DC most of the groups mentioned here and many others met monthly at the Global AIDS Roundtable, which was convened by the Washington DC–based advocacy organization the Global Health Council. Notably, the membership of the Global AIDS Roundtable encompassed dozens of organizations and, predictably, many of them did not (and do not) share the activist orientation of Health GAP and its usual campaign partners. Yet these organizations also clearly were having an impact in Washington during the Bush presidency. Most prominent among these groups, because of its high-profile founder, is DATA (Debt, AIDS, Trade, Africa), founded by U2 lead singer Bono. Even before moving into AIDS, Bono had advocated strongly for debt relief, and now he put his star power to work lobbying a host of powerful politicians, most famously ultraconservative Senator Jesse Helms. He also launched a "Heart of America Tour" on world AIDS Day through the Midwest, with celebrities including Ashley Judd, Chris Tucker, and Lance Armstrong. They visited concert venues, campuses, and churches, generating postcards and phone calls from key Congressional districts and White House constituencies. And so, in the same week that the administration observed activists chained together and "dying" in front of the White House gates, calls and cards reiterating the message were streaming in.

There was still another group of organizations within the Roundtable, exemplified by the Christian relief and development organization World Vision. These groups constituted another remarkable development within the AIDS advocacy landscape—the active participation of evangelical Christian churches and organizations. The engagement of this set of actors, not surprisingly, has been fraught with complexity. These groups, which include the National Association of Evangelicals (NAE) and Billy Graham's organization, Samaritan's Purse, were some of the same groups that reacted to the initial domestic epidemic in the United States with intonations about AIDS being God's punishment of homosexuals.

Further, even now, there are obviously stark differences between these groups and the wider AIDS community about policy approaches to the pandemic, particularly regarding prevention. Most AIDS activists adhere to a harm reduction philosophy of prevention. This philosophy promotes behavior changes that can minimize the negative effects of a potential risky action, such as having sex or using injection drugs. Harm reductionists want to have a spectrum of options available to people to protect themselves, including condoms for sexually active people and clean needles for injection drug users. Most evangelical groups involved in global AIDS advocacy are proponents of abstinence as prevention policy, believing that it is the root behavior itself—sex outside of monogamous marriage or injection drug use—that is the core problem.

This obvious difference between the two groups tends to obscure a more subtle one—the difference between the human rights–based approach embraced by most treatment activists and the charity approach at least implicitly offered by most evangelical groups. The difference manifests itself not only in the prevention debate between the two sides but in the whole approach to AIDS as a social issue. One side believes that treatment, as well as sexual and reproductive choices, information, and freedom from discrimination regardless of life choices or circumstances are *rights* which everyone should enjoy and which the state is obligated to provide. The other side holds that some or all of these types of individual freedom are *privileges*, and in conditions of scarcity or moral danger should be rationed according to some calculus of who is most deserving. And yet, despite these competing ideologies, there has been some common ground on two issues: the urgency of providing treatment, and the obligation of rich nations to provide much more money to make this happen. Like Senator Helms, who later reported being moved by Bono's argument that the Bible contained 2,002 passages instructing us to help each other,[19] many of these organizations now spoke of the compassionate example of Jesus, arguing that the United States was morally obligated to help ameliorate the suffering in Africa.

The confluence of these influences would be clearly seen on January 28, 2003. On that night President George W. Bush took to the stage, in this case a podium in the U.S. House of Representatives, to deliver the annual State of the Union address. Everyone in the chamber and watching on television knew that this year's State of the Union address would be a historic one, because Bush would be making his case to the nation, and by extension to the world, for invading Iraq and toppling the regime of Saddam Hussein. As expected, Bush did focus the second half of his address on the crimes of Saddam against the people of Iraq and their neighbors and on the threat his regime posed to the United States and its allies. Far less expected, however, was the cornerstone of the first half of Bush's speech: the need for the United States to provide treatment to combat AIDS in Africa, where the epidemic had created a humanitarian disaster.

"AIDS can be prevented. Antiretroviral drugs can extend life for many years. And the cost of those drugs has dropped from $12,000 a year to under $300 a year—which places a tremendous possibility within our grasp. Ladies and gentlemen, seldom has history offered a greater opportunity to do so much for so many," said Bush. "We have confronted, and continue to confront, HIV/AIDS in our own country," continued the president. "And to meet a severe and urgent crisis abroad, tonight I propose the Emergency Plan for AIDS Relief—a work of mercy beyond all current international efforts to help the people of Africa."

The plan Bush outlined was designed to prevent seven million new HIV infections, provide access to antiretroviral drugs to at least two million people with AIDS, and provide care and support to ten million people infected and affected by HIV. He then called upon Congress to appropriate $15 billion dollars, including $10 billion in new funds, over the next five years. "This nation can lead the world in sparing innocent people from a plague of nature," Bush concluded, before turning to the need to confront and defeat "the man-made evil of international terrorism."

The State of the Union speech marked a stark change in administration rhetoric. As a presidential candidate, Bush had blithely argued that almost everything that happened in Africa lay outside the circle of American national interest. As president, Bush had demonstrated no particular concern about AIDS or about the poor and marginalized populations that bore the brunt of the epidemic. Yet the pledge of $15 billion represented a 150-fold increase over the Clinton administration's first large grant of $100 million, which followed the ACT UP zaps of the Gore presidential campaign. And it marked a major milestone: the U.S. government at the highest level possible and in the highest profile setting possible had committed itself to providing HIV treatment for people in developing countries.

Less than three months later, on April 29, Bush gave a speech in the White House East Room offering his support for the bipartisan Hyde-Lantos Bill, which would serve as the authorizing vehicle for the proposed $15 billion dollar plan. Ambitiously named the U.S. Leadership Against HIV/AIDS, Tuberculosis, and Malaria Act of 2003, the bill was passed by a 375-41 vote in the House and by voice vote in the Senate, and was signed into law on May 27, 2003. By that time, the cynicism among activists that had temporarily been abated by the large dollar commitments originally cited in the State of the Union address was returning, as the expected battle lines began to reemerge between activists and their opponents.

As the plan for the President's Emergency Plan for AIDS Relief (PEPFAR) began to take shape, a number of fault lines opened up around prevention, finances, and treatment. In the prevention realm, a predictable battle loomed around the administration's decision to adopt the widely hailed Ugandan "ABC" model for prevention. Within this model, "A" stands for "abstinence," "B" for "Be faithful," and "C" for "condom use." Although almost everyone agreed that all are useful tools in an AIDS prevention arsenal, strong disagreements arose over what should be emphasized. Conservatives in the House were able to add an amendment requiring that at least a third of the money spent on prevention go to abstinence-only programs, to the dismay of most AIDS advocates, who argued that such programs were dangerous and not even applicable for many target groups, including women engaged in survival sex work and monogamous women who already *are* faithful within marriage but cannot compel their partners to be, and would lead to wasted resources. Several financial issues also quickly emerged. The first was around the amount of money that would be spent in the first year of the program—with activists arguing that at least a fifth of the five-year sum should be spent in the first year due to the dire circumstances recipient countries were in, while the administration argued for a slower scale-up. In addition, even more contentious was the split of that money between the new bilateral initiative and the already-existing multilateral Global Fund. Activists argued for a 50-50 split, but were deeply disappointed by bilateralists in both the administration and Congress who offered only $200 million as an initial contribution to the Global Fund for the year.

Finally, another front quickly emerged along familiar lines—treatment policy. In Bush's initial State of the Union address, he had triumphantly noted (almost as if it were a success of U.S. government policy rather than a development the government had attempted to thwart at every turn) the drastic downward trajectory of prices for AIDS treatment. He had further noted that these deep reductions had made the possibility of dramatic treatment expansion possible—and these comments had certainly been noticed by activists, who had hoped that they signaled a willingness on the part of the U.S. government to procure these less expensive generic drugs for the new program. These hopes began to wither, however, with the July 2 announcement of Bush's appointee for running the new program. Bush named Randall Tobias, former CEO of drug company Eli Lilly, as Coordinator for International HIV/AIDS Assistance (an ambassador-level position) within the State Department. Activists voiced fears that the former leader of a leading brand-name pharmaceutical company would not be in favor of using government money to buy generic medications for the new program. They also pointed to the fact that Eli Lilly was a leading Republican campaign contributor. The defining battle on the issue of generic medicines would come later, in March 2004, when the administration would convene a meeting in Botswana where it would come out strongly against the purchase of generic "fixed dose combination" drugs that had been approved through a process created by the WHO. But even by the date of Tobias' appointment, a picture of opposing views began to emerge. On the one hand, the administration viewed the PEPFAR—with its emphasis on fourteen (later fifteen) heavily affected countries, its enthusiasm for abstinence- and faith-based organizations to carry out its programming, and on discounted (but still more expensive than generic) brand-name drugs—as the primary vehicle for conducting its global AIDS policy. On the other, activists were fighting for two goals: first, to reestablish the multilateral Global Fund as at least an equal recipient for the U.S. funding streams and, second, to alter elements of the PEPFAR that they viewed as inefficient or even counterproductive in target countries.

A BIGGER AND BOLDER VISION: THE '04 STOP AIDS CAMPAIGN

Although many activists devoted considerable energy in trying to contain the new presidential initiative, which was unfolding in some ways that were decidedly at odds with the initially envisioned Presidential AIDS Initiative promoted by activists, some turned to an emerging political opportunity that had served them so well in the past—a presidential election. The circumstances this time were markedly different—now Bush was running as an incumbent, and the real question was who within the tightly packed field of Democratic hopefuls would emerge as his challenger. In spring of 2003 Health GAP began to circulate the idea among allied groups of putting together a comprehensive AIDS platform to promote among the candidates seeking the presidency. The platform would go beyond treatment to incorporate other important AIDS-related demands, and throughout the spring of 2003 many AIDS, development, and human rights groups con- tributed to its formation. The document that emerged as the result of numerous conference calls hosted by Health GAP and solicitations for input on listserves had nine basic planks, with detailed explanations for each of them. These planks included a specific call for $30 billion by 2008 (essentially a doubling of U.S. promises to that point), support for trade policies that would ensure access to generic medicines, and a host of other demands on the "wish list" of the larger global AIDS movement.

The groups that had been key players in the "platform development," particularly Health GAP and the Global AIDS Alliance, actively recruited endorsements from as broad a spectrum of groups as possible. The national offices of the Presbyterian, United Methodist, and Unitarian Universalist churches all signed, as did the National Organization of Women. In all, more than 200 local, national, and international groups from twenty-five states and twenty-eight countries gave their endorsement.

Although the inspiration for this new set of actions, dubbed the '04 Stop AIDS Campaign, came from the previous Gore zaps, the task before the activists was very different. With the Gore zaps, the primary goal had been to shame Gore about a particular policy position enough to change it. In this case, the goal was to attempt to extract the most progressive global AIDS platform possible as a campaign promise from as many of those individuals running for the Oval Office as possible. This would require several things: first, the candidates needed to become familiar with the dimensions of the problem and the solutions they were being asked to pledge to pursue. But they must not only agree to the specifics of the problem and its solution: they must also internalize its importance as an issue and elevate its salience in the race.

In one sense, this work was easier than the Gore zaps had been. Especially during the initial phases of the race, campaigners did not need to be parti- cularly confrontational. Rather, they needed only to employ the simple technique of "bird-dogging"—that is, of asking coordinated public questions of the candidates to get them acquainted with the issues and on record with their responses. For this work, a new set of actors were deployed—students who lived in and around key early primary and caucus states, particularly New Hampshire and Iowa. To recruit and ready the students for their task, Health GAP, SGAC, and the Global AIDS Alliance staff and volunteers visited campuses with students who had already expressed interest in AIDS issues through participation in SGAC or other AIDS organizations. One team traveled to a large number of schools in the Northeast and Midwest and, later, to conferences and other venues where sympathetic "bird-doggers" might be recruited. Working with whoever showed up at a gathering, the team would present a teach-in. The first half would be a substantive presentation, designed to familiarize audiences with global AIDS as an issue and the platform, as well as offering a small "history lesson" about AIDS activism and the success of the Gore zaps. Then the audience would take part in a role play, trying their hand at crafting questions and asking questions of "Senator Aim-Low" (usually played with memorable zeal by Health GAP staffer Paul Davis). Students learned all kinds of tricks, from making sure to be the first in line at the microphone to holding on tightly to the hand of the candidate when shaking hands until the questioned posed was answered.

These trained students went on the campaign trail to pose their questions, beginning in New Hampshire and Iowa and fanning out to other early primary states. Later, as the candidates began to respond but hesitated to make specific pledges, the questions were supplemented with demonstrations at campaign headquarters in Missouri and Vermont. In Iowa, where the Global AIDS Alliance had more connections, students and faith-based organizations pushed the candidates to sign a pledge indicating their support of all nine planks of the platform. Domestic AIDS activists, with leadership from the New York City–based organizations CHAMP and Housing Works, also joined in with a set of U.S.-based demands, called the AIDS Vote Platform.

By World AIDS Day all the Democratic candidates had taken the pledge and most had unveiled at least some of the platform planks, most commonly the promises of $30 billion and debt cancellation, on their Web sites and in their press statements. However, they continued to resist making AIDS a top-shelf issue, and once the races were over in Iowa (January 19) and New Hampshire (January 27), a window of opportunity began to close. The candidates were dropping out, and small meet-and-greets at local bookstores and middle school libraries had been almost completely replaced by rallies in gymnasiums and auditoriums that offered far less possibility for personal contact and questioning of the candidates. Disruptive tactics—from the milder shouting out a question to the more extreme possibilities like drowning out a candidate's speech with chanting—remained as options but carried a number of tactical and strategic downsides. Not only was the pool of participants willing to volunteer for these higher-risk activities significantly smaller, but they also required much more planning and co-ordination. Furthermore, as it became increasingly apparent that Kerry was the presumptive nominee, attention shifted to the problem of injecting AIDS into the National Party Conventions and the general election. Activists continued to attend events for Senators Kerry and Edwards, but many efforts were increasingly drawn to the opportunities which would present themselves in the summer, namely the upcoming 15th International AIDS Conference to be held in Bangkok, Thailand, and the National Party Conventions for the Democrats and Republicans to be held in Boston and New York City respectively.

Of course, in the interim, there were other struggles being waged, one of which concerned the way that the treatment side of the PEPFAR was evolving. Initially, activists took heart from Bush's own choice of words in his State of the Union address, where he had noted that drug prices had plummeted, making treatment a possibility. Given that the prices he quoted were of generic drugs, there seemed to have been at least an implicit acceptance of their place in the new initiative. Importantly, a number of NGOs were already using them on the ground, and reported especially the promise of "fixed dose combinations" (FDCs), which allowed the combination of two or three drugs into one pill, making compliance with treatment regimens much simpler. But in February, when the government began issuing grants, recipients were unclear on whether the money could be used to buy generic medications. Then the United States began circulating a proposal calling for drug approval standards that would not accept the existing WHO certification process used for these drugs and therefore rule out the purchase of these FDCs. It called for a meeting in late March in Gabarone, Botswana, to consider this proposal.

Predictably, a major controversy arose. Besides the obvious advantage of lower costs, proponents of FDCs argued for the procurement of FDCs with PEPFAR money for another reason as well—simplicity for overburdened and understaffed health care systems. To ask these countries to have different treatment regimens in place—one for PEPFAR recipient groups, one for groups not under PEPFAR restrictions—was seen as burdensome and confusing.

The U.S. government based its position on the issue on regulatory safety. The FDCs had been approved through a process undertaken by the WHO known as "prequalification" but were not FDA approved. Barring such approval, it argued, they could not in good conscience, offer the drugs to Africans. The debate over FDCs was highly significant for several reasons. First, on a practical level, it meant a major difference in how many people could be treated. Additionally, it was viewed as an issue of sovereignty, both in the sense that the United States was asserting itself over the multilateral World Health Organization, and in the sense that it was trampling on the standards of the countries where PEPFAR was operating that had already accepted these pills

Outside the United States, many weren't buying the U.S. position. Among the leaders of the opposition was MSF, which argued that it had been steadily providing data about the efficacy, safety, and quality of FDCs but felt that the U.S. administration was "moving the goal posts every time a particular concern has been addressed."[20] Also at the Botswana meeting one of the four major awardees of PEPFAR money, the Catholic Relief Services Consortium, testified that many lives would be needlessly lost because of the proposed purchasing restrictions. The European community made its annoyance with the U.S. position clear when the European Agency for Medicinal Products, the largest drug regulatory agency in the European Union, simply decided not to send any representatives to the Botswana meeting.

Within the United States, activists went into action in the halls of Congress and in the streets. Within Congressional offices, they lobbied members in both chambers and on both sides of the aisles. Significantly, one of the consequences of their work was letters to the president. The first was written by U.S. Congressman Henry Waxman, a key ally of AIDS activists on a variety of treatment issues. The second reminded him of his own State of the Union speech referencing what could have only been generic medications (given the $300 price he cited) and urged him to allow the purchase of drugs that had been "prequalified" by the WHO. The letter was signed by six senators, including Ted Kennedy and John McCain. Three days after the letter from the senators was sent, AIDS activists led a protest in front of the offices of the drug company lobby PhARMA, where eight people participated in civil disobedience and were arrested.

The administration had its own defenders as well, however, who promoted a different view in the op-ed pages of American newspapers. Leading off was Abner Mason, executive director of the AIDS Responsibility Project and a Bush appointee to the Presidential Advisory Council on HIV/AIDS, who supported the administration's decision in a piece entitled "The False Promise of Untested AIDS Drugs" in the *San Francisco Chronicle*. He was followed by the Manhattan Institute's Robert Goldberg's op-ed in the *Washington Times* which accused FDC proponents of attempting "to force the United States to spend every dime of its $15 billion AIDS initiative on this deadly dose." Next was James K. Glassman, who accused the president's critics of "imperiling millions of Africans" who "deserve respect, not treatment with drugs unfit for the West."[21]

The Botswana meeting concluded with consensus on at least a couple of points, namely that FDCs are a crucial component in the fight against AIDS, and that there should be broadly stated principles that could be used to drive development and approval of the combinations. However, the United States continued its opposition to the standards used by the WHO to prequalify both single dose and combination dose ARVs. And in the months ahead, opponents of the FDCs would find opportunities to continue to press their case.

PRESIDENTIAL PROTESTS IN SUMMER 2004

In planning meetings of activists throughout the late winter and early spring it was becoming clear that many progressive activists promoting a wide range of causes were planning to be on hand for protests at the Republican National Convention slated to be held in late August. As the activists involved in '04 Stop AIDS plotted ways to distinguish themselves from the sea of actions that were being planned, another call for action made its way to the United States from across the Atlantic. South Africa's TAC put out a call to activists worldwide, but especially those within the United States, to take part in a global day of protest against the global AIDS policies of Bush. At issue were both the failure to live up to the $15 billion over five years promise of the State of Union address, and the perceived inefficiencies, such as abstinence-based prevention policies and insistence that money not be spent on generic fixed dose combination drugs, in the money that had been spent.

A number of conference calls were held to decide how to supplement the protests TAC was holding in Cape Town and Johannesburg, and various global groups were planning in Thailand, Kenya, and a number of European cities. American activists decided to hold simultaneous protests at Bush-Cheney headquarters across the country. All of them were to follow a common formula—a protest rally followed by the ceremonial destruction of a common giant voided check for $15 billion. On June 24 there were actions in Seattle; New York City; Lansing, Michigan; Arlington, Virginia; Manchester, New Hampshire; and Cleveland and Columbus, Ohio. The largest protest was held in Harrisburg, Pennsylvania, where some participants of the demonstration, many of whom had made the trip from Philadelphia as members of ACT UP, decided to try to deliver their ripped-up check. On entering the office in order to offer the campaign workers the pieces of cardboard, they found the staff hiding under desks and behind furniture as if under attack.

A little over two weeks later, many activist leaders packed their bags and headed off to Bangkok, Thailand, for the International AIDS Conference, armed with an ambitious to-do list of actions. One of the most important plans was to provide international support and solidarity to Thai activists intent on using the International Conference as an opportunity to shame the Thai government for its deadly policy of "zero-tolerance" for drug use, which had resulted in the extrajudicial execution of approximately 2,600 men, women, and children and the driving underground of drug-using risk behavior.[22]

But closer to home was also a target-rich environment. In the lead-up to the meeting, reports from several newspapers suggested that the administration, still smarting from the protest that had drowned out Tommy Thompson's speech in Barcelona, had found a way to exact its pound of flesh. Whereas in 2002, the U.S. government sent 236 of its scientists to Barcelona, in 2004 the number was dropped to 50 and overall funding for the meeting went from $3.6 million to $500,000. As a result, forty presentations had to be withdrawn and at least three satellite sessions cancelled entirely. Most tellingly, even some scientists with outside funding, such as Marc Bulterys, who works for the CDC but whose trip was being sponsored by the American Medical Association, were simply denied permission to attend. The denial prompted Catherine DeAngelis, editor of the prestigious *Journal of the American Medical Association,* to renounce the U.S. government's actions as "an incredible example of political pettiness."[23] In answer to defenders who argued that the decision was merely a cost-cutting measure, critics pointed out that the same standards seemed not to have applied to Secretary Thompson's December trip to five African countries that cost nearly half a million dollars, including $400,000 for a chartered plane and $10,000 for the services of a public relations firm. Additionally, activists planned to use the occasion to target the Bush administration, both individually for PEPFAR policies emphasizing abstinence and refusing to procure generic fixed dose combination drugs, and collectively as one of the G8 leaders who was supplying insufficient financial support to the Global Fund.

At the opening ceremony, Thai Prime Minister Thaksin Shinawatra's kickoff speech was heckled with catcalls, whistles, and a banner proclaiming "Thaksin lies," and followed up with a roundly critical speech by Paisan Suwannawong, head of the Thai Drug Users Network and Chair of the Thai Treatment Action Group. Among the many protests held were an opening-day protest organized by Thai activists with broad support from other international colleagues under the theme "access for all" and highlighting global gaps in access to both treatment and prevention and a mock trial of the leaders of the industrialized nations who were "convicted" of failure to live up to their countries' commitments to provide $10 billion a year to the Global Fund.

One unexpected development of the conference was the emergence of counterprotesters, apparently affiliated with the group Bureaucrash, which bills itself as being "an international network of activists" opposed to "bloated sprawling governments and the bureaucrats and politicians who control them."[24] The youths involved filmed their action at a protest convened by American, Thai, and other activists against a proposed Thai-U.S. Free Trade Agreement. According to their own account posted, along with their film, on the Web site "Bureaucrash," the student "crashers" moved from their plan to silently hand out flyers to actively mounting their own protest against the Thai and American activists. In answer to the chants from activists to "treat the people, break the patents," they responded with the same message that was emblazoned on their T-shirts: "socialism kills, capitalism heals." Although Health GAP volunteer Allison Dinsmore recalled that they didn't seem very conversant with the issues of AIDS or medicines or trade, they did seem to focus primarily on actions where drug companies were targeted, and reported (also on the Bureaucrash Web site) a second counterprotest in defense of the drug company GlaxoSmithKline.[25]

The opponents of the treatment activists also made use of a news story that had broken shortly before the Bangkok meeting, on May 27. The news was that the WHO had removed two antiretroviral drugs from its prequalification list. To treatment activists, this was merely proof of what they had been saying all along—that WHO standards were sufficiently stringent and vigilant to monitor the safety of the drugs in question. Specifically, they noted that the reason for pulling the drugs was not that the drugs themselves had been shown to be unsafe, but merely that the firm that had been hired to conduct the bioequivalence tests on the drugs had been unable to produce some necessary documentation when the WHO had made a site visit.[26] But opponents of FDCs during the Botswana meeting lost no time in capitalizing on this development. Abner Mason put together a "Petition for Safe Drugs" to be released at a press conference on Tuesday, July 12, the day the Bangkok meeting had designated as focusing on scaling up access to treatment. It made demands on both Cipla (maker of the two drugs delisted) and the WHO to, among other things, run new clinical trials on their products and warrant that all prequalified drugs have the same safety and effectiveness as those approved by developed country regulators, because, in his words, "the world's poor deserve more than false hope and false medicine."

The activists who attended the Bangkok meeting had little more than a month to prepare for what would prove to be the most memorable of all the summer's activities—an action that would be dubbed "the Naked Truth." Within the jam-packed array of progressive causes eager to get their case before the national television cameras in New York City to cover the Republican Convention, AIDS activists conferenced to envision an action that would rise to the top of the media stack. The action they settled on was attention grabbing in two ways: first, it did not have to compete with other actions occurring during the convention because it was done four days before the convention began, on August 25. Second, and more crucially it could not fail to be noticed because the activists carrying it out weren't wearing clothes. In lieu of their clothing, they sported messages painted on their backs and stomachs that read "drop the debt" and "stop AIDS." A string of about a dozen people led by ACT UP stood together on Eighth Avenue in front of the convention site chanting with linked arms, bringing traffic to a standstill. While amazed onlookers stared, several other activists climbed on top of a parked rig to unfurl a large banner with similar messages. They maintained their positions for about ten minutes, plenty of time to be captured in many photos broadcast to local and national media, before being arrested by police.

Less than a week later, on September 1, the "Naked Truth" squad took their protest into the halls of the convention itself. Given the extremely tight precautions taken by organizers to prevent any supporters into the convention building, this was quite a feat. The activists, many of whom had been personally involved in the previous action on Eighth Avenue, managed to obtain seats within the audience of the Youth Convention, which was to be addressed by first President Bush's daughters and then White House Chief of Staff Andrew Card. The activists waited through the Bush twins' speech and then ripped off their dress shirts to reveal T-shirts bearing the message "Bush Lies. Stop AIDS. Drop the Debt Now," unfurled a banner with a similar message, and began a chant of "Bush Lies" and "Fight AIDS Now" to drown out Card's words. The action was greeted with anger on the convention floor, with young Republicans rushing at the protestors and at least one young man caught on camera by the local news kicking one of the student protestors. Although both protests garnered coverage in the media, neither had the desired effect on the incumbent candidate. The Republican National Convention rolled on, with no serious discussion of upping commitments or changing policies in directions remotely favored by global (or domestic) AIDS activists.

TWO STEPS FORWARD, ONE STEP BACK

After the Republican National Convention, the political pulse of the country quickened, as partisans on both sides geared up for an election that was widely seen as being determined by the side most able to mobilize its true believers. For the vast majority of people heavily involved with both domestic and international AIDS advocacy, there was a palpable fear of another four-year term under the Bush administration. On a wide variety of AIDS-related fronts, it seemed increasingly apparent that AIDS policies at home and abroad were converging. From the growing trend to grant AIDS service contracts to faith-based organizations with Evangelical Christian ties, to the perceived antagonism against biological and social scientists conducting research on a wide variety of topics, especially ones focusing around human sexuality, to the elevation of abstinence-only prevention programs above other forms of prevention work: in all these areas, directives from government aimed at both U.S. citizens and foreign aid recipients were becoming increasingly congruent.

Frustration had also been building on the treatment side of the equation on the domestic front. Clearly the treatment situation in the United States is not as appallingly tragic as it is in most developing countries. But it is appalling in its own right to note that in the richest country in the world, hundreds of people are sitting on waiting lists, with their only chance for treatment coming from the death of a fellow citizen currently being treated whose place they can assume. An analysis conducted by the Kaiser Family Foundation released in December 2004 found that even after distribution of a supplemental $20 million to bolster failing ADAP programs, more than 800 remained on waiting lists.[27] Furthermore, these lists count only those people who are financially eligible, not the numbers (possibly in the thousands) of uninsured or underinsured individuals whose incomes are too high for the AIDS Drug Assistance Program criteria within their states, but too low to afford to buy their medications. Additionally, these numbers do not reflect the many cost-cutting measures that states make, including reducing the list of drugs they will provide, that affect the quality of treatment.

Yet another obvious common frustration with treatment in developing countries and the United States for AIDS activists has been the power of the brand-name pharmaceutical companies to control prices of the drugs. In developing countries this has mainly played out with the brand-name companies using their influence to create multilateral and bilateral agreements for patent protections to keep generic competition out, and in a pinch, offering deep discounts to stave off demands for the generics. In the United

States, these same companies charge, in many if not most cases, the most expensive prices in the world, and use their influence in Congress to ward off any price control measures. An extreme example of this occurred with the drug Ritonavir marketed by Abbott Laboratories under the trade name Norvir. Ritonavir was developed with federal money—a multimillion dollar grant from the National Institutes of Health, and it is marketed by Abbott not as it was originally developed (that is, as a protease inhibitor) but rather as a booster to heighten the effects of other protease inhibitors. Although Abbott's investment in clinical trials is estimated at under $15 million, its sales of Norvir totaled $1 billion during its first five years in the market (1996–2001).[28] Despite the seemingly obvious profitability of the drug, in December 2003, Abbott increased the private sector price (though not the Medicaid or ADAP price) of Norvir 400 percent, pushing the cost of the most common booster dose (200 mg) from $1,600 per year to $7,800. It did not increase the cost of its own Kaletra product, however, which meant that the cost of competitor drugs that use Norvir as a booster would go up, but its own product containing a booster dose would gain a competitive edge. A broad coalition of doctors and domestic AIDS activists around the country mobilized to bring press coverage to Abbott's action and petition the government to exercise its "march in" authority stemming from a law known as the Bayh-Dole Act that would allow the Secretary of Health and Human Services to open competition on a patent that was developed with federal funding. Although both Congress and the National Institutes of Health held hearings on the issue, the government ultimately refused to act. Explaining the NIH's August 4, 2004, ruling, director Elias Zerhouni claimed, "The issue of drug pricing has global implications and thus, is appropriately left for Congress to address legislatively."[29]

The convergence of Bush administration policy approaches regarding its domestic and global agendas helped domestic and international activists find common cause in their hopes that a more progressive administration might replace the incumbent. But that failed to happen in November 2004, when to the great dismay of the vast majority of the global treatment activist movement, the Bush administration was reelected for a second term. Although it was considered a great setback by treatment activists and the larger allied AIDS movement, it was hardly a new situation. The first wave of AIDS treatment activism rose up in the face of a presidential administration that the movement considered antithetical to its goals, and indeed to the very existence of much of its membership. The situation is now somewhat more complex, since the U.S.-based portion of the global AIDS treatment movement must balance the political circumstances within its own country with the external politics and opportunities outside its borders.

But many of treatment activism's greatest victories have paradoxically come at the times of its greatest political challenges, and it would not be surprising if the movement is able to forge a vibrant strategy to fit its new circumstances. In the Conclusion and Afterword by Health GAP founder Alan Berkman, we take a last look at these challenging decisions facing the movement.

Conclusion

The two AIDS treatment activist movements described in this book—the first domestic, the second global—have obvious links and parallels. The first, launched in March 1987 by the radical new activist group ACT UP, followed a call-to-arms speech by Larry Kramer. Very quickly it orchestrated an angry, attention-grabbing protest on Wall Street calibrated to achieve maximum exposure for its primary demands of new and affordable drugs and its related calls for prevention education, rights protection, and political leadership. The second U.S.-based movement also began its actions in the spring, in this case in 1999, after being brought together by Alan Berkman for the purpose of dramatically increasing treatment access around the globe. As with the earlier movement this one began with a face-off against a powerful opponent—the U.S. Congress, which was bent on passing the African Growth and Opportunities Act. This project was followed by the one that would literally put it all over the map, beginning in Carthage, Tennessee. There, Al Gore's kickoff event announcing his candidacy in the 2000 presidential race quickly descended into every politician's nightmare as activists blew whistles, waved banners, and chanted. With relentless doggedness, activists would follow him on the campaign trail, disrupting events and demanding "AIDS Drugs for Africa."

Perhaps it is no coincidence that both movements began in spring, the season of birth and renewal. Certainly, both also experienced a conceptual springtime of sorts in the form of "cognitive liberation." As we have discussed throughout this book, cognitive liberation is that essential spark that inspires the members of a movement with the conviction that a situation is wrong, that it could possibly be changed, and that they as individuals and as a group can help to make it right (or at least improve it). For the first domestic movement, this understanding came from a personal place, as community members experienced the rage and frustration of watching their own partners and friends fall sick and die in pain heightened by a sense of both futility, as the community waited in vain for effective treatments, and oppression, as society more commonly responded to the problem with blame and discrimination than with compassion and concern. The idea that this state of affairs could, and indeed must, change was slower in coming, but was helped along by the self-empowerment philosophy that had already created PWA chapters in a number of cities, together with Kramer's serendipitous call for action.

By contrast, the second movement's cognitive kick-start was grounded in empathy and a form of survivor guilt. The empathy felt by the second wave of activists in the United States was a rare occurrence in a world where wealth, health, and other types of disparities between developed and developing nations grow ever starker. But in this case, veterans of the early days of AIDS in the United States actually could empathize with the pain of those in developing countries. Starvation, lack of clean water, civil war, other infectious diseases, and a whole host of other causes of the misery that are so common in so many parts of the planet are almost never directly felt in the United States. AIDS is different. Though AIDS-affected U.S. citizens had never experienced most of the problems facing those in the developing world, they at least had a point of reference with regard to the suffering, death, and grief associated with AIDS. And some experienced a form of survivor guilt because the antiretroviral medications that they had access to were all but unavailable in the developing world. This empathy and survivor guilt led to anger on the part of some activists as they came to understand that wealthy governments and pharmaceutical companies were actively choosing to withhold the ability to access cheap medications and the means for paying for them.

Another commonality was the experience of early success by the domestic and global movements, which set in motion a cycle of positive reinforcement. Early victory is important in the momentum of any new movement, and both were highly successful in that regard. The 1987 Wall Street action by ACT UP achieved a price reduction for AZT, the first medication approved to specifically fight HIV, while the Gore protests resulted in the turnaround of Clinton-Gore trade policy regarding South Africa's ability to procure affordable drugs. Once begun it is clear that both movements were able to translate the key elements of surprise, victory, and heavy media coverage into rapid forward movement.

ONE (GIANT) STEP FORWARD: THE DOMESTIC TREATMENT ACTIVIST MOVEMENT

In taking stock of the first movement we can see both its own major accomplishments and its role as a seedbed for the second globally oriented movement that would follow it. The movement accomplished an enormous amount in the six years between 1987 and 1993. These accomplishments came in two varieties: substantive victories and altered power structures. Topping the list in the first column would have to be the initial demands that brought the movement together in the first place—the rapid development of medications that would treat both HIV and the opportunistic infections that stem from it. That pharmaceutical companies were forced on numerous occasions to lower their prices is also directly attributable, in large degree, to the strenuous and informed actions of this movement. Additional changes resulting largely from this movement include alterations in the ways that clinical trials are conducted, the broadening of access to technical medical information, and even changes in the way that AIDS itself is defined. The public financing of AIDS drugs for many people without insurance, first through state programs and beginning in 1990 through national legislation, is also a tribute to activist work and demands.

Altered power structures, though less obvious to many observers, are an equally important legacy and occurred at a variety of levels. Individuals learned to challenge their health care providers, their service delivery systems, and their communities and to insist that they must have power in the decisions that affected their own lives. As groups, PWA organizations also worked to ensure that they were represented in government policymaking bodies and in conferences and other arenas where information was produced and disseminated. The idea that PWA voices could and should have equal weight at the table for the discussion of everything from the design of clinical trials to the implementation of service programs seems common sense today: yet it was once a radical demand. The mainstreaming of many of these accomplishments and recalibrated power equations is testament to how profoundly the movement was able to impact its targets.

Still another critical power shift came with the understanding (or perhaps more accurately, rediscovery) that there are more sources of power than simply money and social status. Compared with the pharmaceutical corporations, government officials, and health professionals they were targeting, activists were at a severe disadvantage in terms of access to these types of resources. Yet, the activists were able to fill the gap by creatively thinking about the resources they *did* have—excellent skills in framing issues and media work, willingness to be disruptive in systems that feared negative exposure, and compelling moral arguments. By demonstrating their willingness to use all these tools—and to the degree that they were able to withstand co-optation—the activist movement was able to actually *create* power that helped to level the playing field between them and their targets.

Despite significant progress, some domestic treatment victories have also been eroded in recent years. The treatment that had been made available to citizens who were otherwise unable to pay for the expensive antiretroviral combination therapies has been rolled back as financially strapped states have trimmed their AIDS Drug Assistance Programs (ADAPs) and placed people on waiting lists in the push to erect ever-higher barriers to individuals seeking government support. The tacit standoff between domestic AIDS activists and the pharmaceutical industry is also increasingly strained, as skyrocketing domestic prices of AIDS medications in an age of cutbacks on both ADAP and privately financed health care through managed care make drug access more problematic. The December 2003 announcement by Abbott Laboratories of a 400 percent increase in the price of Norvir unleashed a firestorm of criticism from AIDS activists, doctors, and some in Congress. It was, as one Democratic Senator put it, "a nexus of all the bad practices that all the drug companies use."[1] And yet this outrage failed to inspire the federal government to make use of its "march-in" authority that would have allowed the government to challenge the pricing of the drug.

Although this volume has focused on issues related to treatment, it is also important to note that other closely related issues, especially HIV prevention, have also been losing ground in the United States. Indeed, AIDS activists have been more successful in establishing an enduring legacy in the realm of treatment provision than in certain aspects of prevention, such as condom distribution, comprehensive sex education, and sterile syringe exchange. This is ironic considering that the privacy rights inherent in progressive prevention policies have been upheld (at least in some contexts) by U.S. courts, whereas health care is not, and never has been, held to be a right in this country. Since 2001, conservative federal government policies promulgated by the Bush administration and further abetted by an anti-privacy, pro-security ethic in the wake of September 11, have further reversed the gains of AIDS prevention activists. These reversals have important implications for PWA and at-risk communities and, consequently, for the forward-looking agendas of AIDS treatment activists and the larger AIDS advocacy movement.

Another largely unacknowledged problem is that some very important issues have never had much traction to begin with. The epidemic in the United States has been increasingly borne by communities marginalized by race, ethnicity, and income, yet many of the AIDS issues especially important to these communities have never been pushed with the same force as the treatment access agenda; these issues include expansion of addiction treatment programs, provisions of decent HIV/AIDS care and prevention services in correctional facilities, and elimination of immigration laws that discriminate against HIV-positive individuals.

In all, the AIDS activist agenda has been severely undermined by the Bush administration. The harm reduction approach that sought to minimize the effects of risky behavior has been replaced—in dealing with both sexual and drug-using behaviors—with strong advocacy of abstinence, and faith-based organizations instead of public health or secular groups have been increasingly deputized as the bearer of this message. Looking at the current political landscape it appears that the rights-based vision that has always been the foundation of both the domestic AIDS treatment access movement and the larger advocacy movement of which it was part is increasingly besieged by a morality- and charity-based approach by the individuals and institutions that have controlled the federal government since 1990.

THE IMPACT OF GOING GLOBAL

Beyond its policy gains, the first treatment access movement has a second and equally important legacy in that it served as a foundation for the U.S.-based portion of the global treatment access movement that would follow it. The beginning of the global treatment access movement was grafted onto the remaining infrastructure of a handful of surviving ACT UP chapters. Although the initial call bringing various groups together came from outside ACT UP, it was ACT UP that provided the majority of the bodies and tactics for most of the second movement's earliest work. All four of Health GAP's initial staffers came from ACT UP—three from ACT UP Philadelphia and one from ACT UP New York. And the second movement made very heavy use of the strategy and tactics of the first, adopting an insider-outsider strategy that involved a willingness to resort to protest and civil disobedience to raise attention and prompt action. Movement members also developed an ability to come to the table as "amateur experts" for tough negotiation with government officials, pharmaceutical companies, and others. Equally important, the first movement modeled the successful use of information and symbolic politics, showing how good media work could force an issue into mainstream news coverage, and how potent symbols and visuals could get it on the front page. Perhaps most useful of all, the first movement also demonstrated the importance of being willing to constantly "push the envelope" in terms of both the nature and scope of demands, so that what is initially dismissed as utopian eventually becomes widely accepted.

Like the movement from which it descended, the second treatment access movement is remarkable for having achieved a paradigm shift. The first movement redefined people living with a disease from the objects of pity (and sometimes of judgment) to the arbiters of how that disease should be dealt with. That change has affected not only other disease-based groups, who have been inspired to redefine themselves, but also the visions and procedures of government, treatment providers, and researchers. Similarly, the second movement has forced governments, the public health community, and the polity of developed countries to reverse the unquestioned assumption that treatment cannot be provided to the poor. It scored this accomplishment by doing two things. First, on a practical level it blew apart the myth that universal treatment is unaffordable—both by exposing the actual (as opposed to retail) costs of the drugs involved and by showing how small these costs are in relative terms. Second, it countered the prevalent market- and charity-based approaches with a compelling rights-based narrative that had tremendous resonance with many target audiences.

In order to accomplish this goal, the movement had to evolve in a whole new way, however, which was to link up and work in partnership with other domestic movements, international organizations, and passionate individuals across the globe. This forging of the global treatment access network was both critical to successfully overturning the prevailing paradigm and a victory in itself. The network has often linked in imperfect configurations that continued to privilege what treatment activist Gregg Gonsalves has referred to as "secondary activists"—specialists with highly developed skills—over "primary activists"—the mass movement of people putting their bodies on the line in pursuit of their own interests.[2] Although the networking has its flaws, it represents an exciting means of sharing experiences, skills, and passion beyond national boundaries. It can also draw strength from the numbers that can be gathered transnationally, and from the possibilities of pushing targets from a multitude of vantage points.

Tangibly, this transnational movement has not only altered a dominant way of thinking: it has also set in motion mechanisms for achieving an alternative vision. Because of the movement the brand-name pharmaceutical makers have lowered their prices, and on occasion given drugs away. In reality, though, these were never major goals of the movement, and actually have been seen as impediments to the real goal, which has been to force these companies to stop blocking competition from generic companies, which, once unblocked, has the effect of bringing prices down overall. The fact that generic medications, and particularly more easily administered generic multidose combination drugs, are now being bought in many developing countries is the true indicator of success of the global treatment access movement.

That the drugs are being bought also points to a second area of success of the movement. In 1999, when Health GAP was formed, the United States spent no money on AIDS treatment in developing countries and almost none on general AIDS programming. According to the Congressional Research Service, the U.S. Agency for International Development (USAID) spent $81 million on AIDS in Africa in fiscal year 1999, and just $67 million the year before.[3] Less than five years later, the U.S. government was in the midst of unrolling its multibillion dollar PEPFAR initiative with a stated goal of putting two million people into treatment. And the Global Fund to Fight AIDS, Tuberculosis, and Malaria that had been launched in January 2002 at the behest of UN Secretary General Kofi Annan had disbursed billions of dollars to individual countries that had submitted proposals for addressing their critical AIDS, tuberculosis, and malaria needs. Although there are major continuing deficiencies and implementation problems with both these programs, they represent monumental leaps forward compared with the apathy that preceded them.

THE GLOBAL MOVEMENT AT A CROSSROADS

The U.S.-based global treatment access movement stands at a crossroads. Its members are considering the implications of two major developments, one of their own making, the other the result of outside actors. The first of these is the actual success of the movement. Although it is certainly true that the ultimate goal—universal treatment access—is not even close to having been achieved, major steps have been taken in that direction. According to the Keck and Sikkink model, a transnational activist network can succeed in any of five ways: by framing debates and getting issues on the agenda, encouraging commitments from states and other actors, creating procedural change, affecting policy, and changing the behavior of others. To greater and lesser degrees, all of these have happened as the result of the global treatment access movement (and before it, as the result of the domestic one).

As noted above, the success of these movements in the first area, framing debates, has been nothing short of remarkable. Today, to suggest withholding treatment in developing countries to preserve all the money for prevention seems reprehensible. Yet at the advent of the global treatment access movement this was precisely the position of almost all the players in positions to make decisions on this issue—international organizations, wealthy donor countries led by the United States, and most public health experts in the global North. The complete nature of this paradigm shift is testament to the success of the movement. Although far short of the need, the commitments activists were able to wring from both the U.S. government and the United Nations countries for the PEPFAR and the Global Fund respectively also have no parallel in other health issues.

At the same time that activists around the world take some satisfaction in the gains they have achieved, their attention is also focused on an external development—the consolidation of domestic and global AIDS policy by the U.S. government. Particularly in the past two years, it is hard to escape the conclusion that the Bush approaches to global and domestic AIDS are increasingly congruent. Domestically, treatment in the United States has always privileged intellectual property protection over affordability, which is why the United States has the most highly priced drugs in the world. At least until recently, the government has been able to maintain at least a tacit stalemate on the issue by using ADAPs to make otherwise-unaffordable drugs available to those who need them. But as ADAPs run dry, this makeshift solution will be increasingly untenable. In the global realm, the idea of simple drug distribution is even more unrealistic. This is why the generic drug debate has been so much more vigorously fought by the second treatment access movement than the first. The U.S. government's position in both cases—to side with the brand-name pharmaceuticals domestically and globally (even when it is literally standing against the rest of the world)—shows no sign of shifting.

On the prevention front, the harmonization is equally pronounced. Globally and domestically, the U.S. government has been clear that it favors a simplistic prevention message of "abstinence until monogamous heterosexual marriage," and that it sees faith-based organizations as ideally placed to deliver it (and to be given federal funds for doing so). Recently the United States has also sought to export its domestic animosity to harm reduction approaches, such as by opposing any international support for sterile syringe distribution or needle exchange programs and by requiring recipients to explicitly repudiate, and thus stigmatize, sex work. The net result is that more vulnerable people are likely to become infected as prevention strategies become less geared to the realities of their life circumstances.

These moves are forcing U.S. activists in the global treatment access movement to make some tough decisions. Do these developments mean that activists should go more "broad and shallow" by picking up new issues in addition to treatment and/or by deliberately forging more far-ranging coalitions with domestic activists, or should they stay "narrow and deep" by focusing on global AIDS treatment only? This is a monumental question, since even the seemingly simpler of the two agendas, staying "narrow and deep," is still ambitious. Major global treatment scale-up will require more funds, better delivery systems, and a massive increase in health care providers, particularly in sub-Saharan Africa. Thus activists will have to push to get more resources to the Global Fund, the treatment-oriented portions of

PEPFAR, and other programs providing treatment. They will also need to advocate for technical assistance and community involvement to improve the treatment delivery within these programs. Helping countries build their own sustainable systems will also require multiple efforts to facilitate access to the cheapest effective drugs, divert money being spent on debt repayment to treatment delivery and other services, and improve the capacity of health systems by improving and increasing the training and compensation of health care professionals as well as the physical facilities in which they work.

The move to broaden the focus of the movement might include focusing on other key AIDS issue areas, including prevention—from condoms to needle exchange to microbicide and vaccine development—and protecting the human rights of those living with and affected by HIV. Treatment activists have always known, and indeed have always argued, that these areas must be pushed in conjunction with treatment, but now the more difficult question is raised as to whether to continue to mainly support allies working in these areas, or delve in directly themselves. Broadening could also mean explicitly taking on the deeper structural causes of the pandemic, such as poverty, unequal effects of globalization, and discrimination against women, sexual minorities, and other marginalized groups. As with the AIDS issue areas mentioned above, the crucial connections between these problems and the goals of both expanding treatment and more broadly eradicating the AIDS pandemic are undeniable. However, each of these issue areas is bound up in cultural and socioeconomic complexities that raise profound challenges, particularly for a small U.S.-based group with limited expertise or experience in these areas. A hallmark of AIDS activists has always been their agility in adapting to new circumstances and acquiring new skills sets, and these are important assets in this consideration. But the question of going "broad and shallow" versus "narrow and deep" remains a difficult one.

FRAMING THE ISSUES

The theoretical frameworks employed in this book offer some insights about these choices, but seem to suggest conflicting paths. McAdam work on the civil rights movement points to a disintegration that was based in a loss of focus, geographically and substantively. As the civil rights movement expanded from its southern local bases to the north and west, it lost strength and connectivity. And as the substance of the goals switched from deseg-regation to incorporate a host of other social justice concerns, McAdam argues, it lost its way, as internal conflicts over direction erupted within the movement. Keck and Sikkink, on the other hand, predicate the success of the movements they examine on precisely the opposite characteristics. To them, the key is to link disparate problems under the same umbrella (so that, for instance, female genital mutilation, bride burning, and domestic violence come together in a common struggle opposing violence against women), and to bring together many far-flung actors.

Another key point within the Keck and Sikkink framework suggests a difficulty the movement will face regardless of which direction it takes—the problem of issue framing. They argue that a key characteristic of a successful issue is that it has a short causal train of responsibility—in simplistic terms, a villain. And both the domestic and global activist movements have been able to frame the treatment issue with this causal train leading in a clear and simple way to an obstructionist adversary. In fact, in both cases they actually began with one prevailing issue narrative: a plea for resources to be distributed to members of unpopular groups to alleviate a stigmatized condition. And both were able to frame the issue as a compelling story of heroes and villains—a brave band of activists coming together for a pitched struggle against a callous, profit-driven pharmaceutical industry being aided by a complicit government in the quest to keep affordable medications out of the hands of dying people.

Whichever road the movement takes, framing the next chapter will be more difficult. If it stays focused on treatment, the issues will become more subtle. Governments and corporations now have talking points to claim they are on the side of the angels—by providing PEPFAR, by agreeing to the Doha Declaration, by offering some treatment to some people. The next generation of activist demands are likely to include the need for treatment rollout to be accelerated, for bilateral trade agreements to be scrutinized as arduously as the big multilateral trade accords, and for fixed dose combination drugs to be prioritized. These more technical questions will be much harder to package in a compelling, good-versus-evil narrative that captures front-page headlines and the imagination of a general audience.

The same basic complication awaits the movement if it moves in a broadening direction. One of the reasons that treatment was able to be such a successful wedge issue for the larger AIDS movement is that it is, by its very nature, compelling. Drugs can be the difference between life and death, and most people are not, in principle, opposed to people having drugs that can save their lives. The same is not true for condoms or clean needles or yet-to-be-developed microbicidal gels or creams. Despite strong scientific evidence, there is no national, let alone global, ideological consensus on the relationship of these prevention tools and HIV transmission. This greatly complicates a causal narrative, and especially the ability to define the target in a political campaign. For instance, is the problem with the governments that refuse to provide the condoms, the men who refuse to use them, or the societies that condone a sexual double standard in marriage? The same is true in work addressing structural changes, which are inherently complex and embedded with obstacles at multiple levels.

Obviously, none of this is to say that the task of framing these new focus issues is impossible, just that framing is critical, and that the next stage in the struggle will necessitate more creative thinking. It may also, at least initially, mean that victories come more slowly and with less fanfare than many of the dramatic changes wrought by the first two treatment activist movements—and this change in pace could also have negative impacts on the movement. Clearly, either path is fraught with significant challenge.

As a practical matter, it appears that the movement is at least leaning in the broadening direction, although there are signs that it is also not giving up on the deepening work, especially with regard to continuing work on trade agreements and on monitoring programs, such as those funded by PEPFAR and the Global Fund, that have been put in place. But even in these areas, the coalitions and issue bases are expanding. Trade agreement activism finds common cause with antiglobalization activists opposed to trade agreements for their negative environmental, labor, and other effects, and activists who are planning monitoring projects are partnering with groups to look at program effects on both treatment and prevention.

Because both treatment access movements have used coalition politics as a key means of achieving their goals, the wishes of their coalition partners are important factors in this decision. And these partners from allied movements, as well as from the Southern corners of the global treatment access movement, see AIDS in much more holistic terms. Northern allied groups that deal with structural problems, such as poverty and gender inequity, are inherently more likely to see the "big picture"—and to push others to it as well—in their work. As for activist partners in the global South, they must live every day not only with the effects of lack of treatment but also with the grinding lack of resources and injustices that make AIDS so common in their communities, and which make the effects of it so much harder to cope with than in the developed world. For them, treatment is critical, but so is the ability for their children to go to school, for their daughters to be able to live to adulthood, and for their families to be able to maintain themselves together after the breadwinners die. In the first wave of the treatment activist movement in the United States, the idea of personal empowerment and the protection of privacy and sexual autonomy was always seen as integral to the work of ACT UP even as it went forward pushing for drug development and affordable prices. Now, if the movement is true to its roots, it must look to the communities it seeks to work in partnership with, to hear from them the specific issues which are integral to making treatment a meaningful contribution to the quality of their lives.

The issue of AIDS treatment has served as an extremely useful opening to bring a host of other issues onto the table. It is possible, for instance, to imagine that there could have been a Global Fund strictly for AIDS, but it is difficult to believe that there could have been the necessary political pressure and subsequent leadership for such a fund strictly for tuberculosis and malaria. Ultimately, it was AIDS activism that ensured that all three major infectious disease killers would finally be addressed, and it is likely that treatment can continue to serve that wedge function, but in conjunction with an expanded array of demands. It will certainly complicate the political work of the movement if it broadens its focus. It may mean, for instance, parting ways with situational allies in and outside of government, who can support the goal of treatment but are not interested in, or actively opposed to, empowering women in their sexual and reproductive choices as a critical AIDS prevention tool.

In a sense, the transition from the first U.S.-based treatment activist movement into the second was itself a broadening of important proportions. The first movement was literally community based, springing from the urban neighborhoods where people perceived a disease wrecking their lives and the lives of the people they cared about. The second movement has succeeded to the extent that people have been able to expand the boundaries in their minds, and the minds of some of the general population, about what constitutes a community, and what it means to belong to one. The global treatment activist movement is motivated by the belief that treatment is the right of everyone, not simply of those in a community defined by shared citizenship or economic status. The success of the next wave of the movement will depend on the ability of activists now to push further and convince people that a whole host of human rights and not *only* treatment should be shared by us all.

Afterword: Realizing Our Victories

Alan Berkman, M.D., Founder of Health GAP

The vision is what unites us: countries supporting each other to build the capacity and commitment to treat every person, adult and child, with HIV; the hope and health that come with treatment strengthening community mobilization to stop the spread of HIV and mitigate its impact; the emotional impact of desperately ill people getting well eroding the wall of stigma that traditionally makes prevention so difficult. Underlying it all, a sense of solidarity that extends throughout populations and across national boundaries.

Drugs into Bodies analyzes the global treatment access movement and chronicles the important progress that it has catalyzed over the past few years. Yet, for all the progress, the constraints of an unequal world, a profit-driven global economy, and antipoor policies continue to create obstacles and set limits that must be overcome. The alliance of poor and developing countries with non-governmental organizations that successfully challenged TRIPS at Doha is now being undermined by heavy-handed efforts by the United States to negotiate regional trade agreements that swap empty promises of economic development for concessions on the protections won at Doha.

Underlying all the successful campaigns of the global treatment access movement is the principle that every human life matters, and that "every" includes people whose choice of partners, drugs, sexual behaviors, and life styles may not (or may) match those of the people who run governments and corporations; we also recognize that many people in the world, particularly poor women, have their choices shaped by poverty, discrimination, and violence. This puts us at odds with the Bush administration's strategy to link treatment with prevention policies that value virginity over life. The treatment access movement has at various times been accused of promoting treatment over prevention; it was never true, but now we must avoid the temptation of supporting government programs that expand treatment while attacking people's right to scientific, lifesaving prevention messages and services. Different organizations may emphasize treatment, prevention, or mitigation, but as a movement, we must be united by a commitment to human rights and social justice or we will have won a battle but lost the war to halt the epidemic.

Much of our energy over the next few years will be spent defending what was won in the years since 1999. Because of those early years, there are now more people with HIV, organizations, and governments mobilized to fight for expanded treatment. Verbal commitments by governments (including those of some of the most heavily impacted countries) and international agencies to expand treatment access have largely resulted in endless policy papers, national plans, and bureaucratic directives—but relatively few people on treatment. "Shame and blame," hopefully an even more effective tactic because of the pronouncements that have been made, will continue to be part of our strategy. Funding commitments to the Global Fund and bilateral programs must be met, effective technical assistance through the WHO and other agencies must be supported and strengthened, and guidelines about the participation of civil society groups, particularly people with HIV, must result in real involvement and leadership at the country and international levels.

UNAIDS and others have said for years that "we know what to do" to control the global epidemic. I fear that there is more than a little hubris in this comment, particularly when we are addressing intimate human behaviors. But we do know some things to do that can save lives, and the challenge is to generate an operational plan and a series of action steps to accomplish them. The World Health Organization's 3×5 and 8×10 plans (8 million on treatment by 2010) are a start, and those goals must be reached. The 3×5 plan was announced in July 2002, but literally nothing of significance happened for more than a year. Three million people died during that year, and we now know that the goal of three million people on treatment was not even approached by the end of 2005. We should recognize the significant steps forward that have been taken, but we should never accept the delays and unnecessary deaths.

We do know some of the policies that must be changed if eight million people are going to have access to lifesaving treatment before the end of the decade. User fees for health care keep poor people from accessing care, and they must be abolished. International financial institutions such as the IMF and World Bank have forced governments to impose these fees in exchange for loans, and many finance ministers in poor countries continue to believe that it is a sound policy. The impact on health care has been disastrous, and there is irony and idiocy in the idea of combating an epidemic while implementing policies that keep people out of care. At the international level, where Health GAP and other international groups have been most effective, the time has come to demand that the international financial institutions change their policy and compensate governments for any revenue shortfall that may result from their termination. Our demand should be for universal free access to treatment. Anything less will continue to marginalize the poor, discriminate against women, and undermine any chance of meeting treatment goals.

When Health GAP was first formed in 1999, we debated whether it was right to focus on AIDS (distinct from TB, malaria, and other treatable diseases), on treatment (distinct from prevention), and on public health (distinct from economic development). At that time, I argued that it was strategic to focus our energies, and that treatment for HIV/AIDS was the wedge issue that could spark a movement and eventually open up the broader discussion of what is needed to control the HIV epidemic and other infectious diseases. Now, the advances that have been made bring us directly up against all these important issues that we self-consciously chose not to focus on in 1999. Keeping people with HIV alive requires controlling TB and malaria; treatment without effective prevention will never control the epidemic; antipoor economic policies perpetuate poverty and inequality and block people from accessing care and treatment. We have now opened the Pandora's box of the world's ills that we always knew was there.

Drugs into Bodies characterizes this moment in the development of the treatment access movement as a time when we must choose between "going deeper" and "going broader." At the individual and organizational level, where time, energy, and expertise are finite, that indeed may be true. For the treatment access movement, though, the strategic question is the same that it's always been: how do we keep "going forward"?

In 1999, the only way we could generate the initial momentum needed to go forward on the global scale was to focus narrowly on AIDS treatment. Now, because of the successes we've had, the only way to go forward as a movement is to go *both* deeper and broader. The conditions that should shape our strategy for the rest of the decade are significantly different than they were in 1999 in a number of ways, as outlined below.

The obstacles and challenges that must be overcome to achieve global treatment access are now much clearer and more concrete. In the past, the United States and other G8 countries dismissed arguments to change IMF and World Bank (and country-level) policies as "merely" ideologically motivated demands from radical groups. Now, they must confront the fact that they will never meet their own goal of universal access by the end of the decade if users' fees remain in place.

Wealthy governments and international agencies have made commitments and set targets, and it is easier to hold them accountable. One of the arguments used by the United States government in the past to oppose global treatment access was that the health care infrastructure in sub-Saharan Africa and other heavily impacted countries was too weak; now, with PEPFAR in place, there are people in the Bush administration and Congress who have a stake in figuring out how to strengthen those systems. This can make "shame and blame" tactics more effective, create the basis for conditional alliances with implementation people within government and international agencies, and open up a political space for the treatment access movement to put forward our own policy proposals for addressing the challenges of delivering quality services in poor and developing countries.

The global treatment access movement is stronger and broader than ever before. The treatment access movement didn't start in 1999. PWA groups in both developed countries and developing countries such as Brazil and Thailand had been active and making demands on their governments for years. The formation of TAC in South Africa, the epicenter of the global epidemic and a high-profile country, and of Health GAP in the United States, the world's only superpower and the home of most of the big pharmaceutical companies, catalyzed the formation of a *global* treatment access movement. In the years since then, PWA groups in many more countries have taken up the demand for HIV treatment. They are the foundation of the movement and make it stronger than it ever has been. The treatment access movement has also broadened its strategic partnerships; in the United States, for example, organizations that traditionally focused on domestic AIDS issues and those focusing on global AIDS issues are increasingly uniting on a common agenda. Similarly, human rights groups, reproductive rights groups, and the treatment access movement will increasingly need to engage in formulating a common agenda or risk a setback to all the work in the current political climate in the United States

If the U.S.-based movement is to avoid the dangers of having to choose between "going deeper" and "going broader," we will need to deepen our alliances with strategic partners and broaden our conception of who constitutes the treatment access movement. We need to move forward and insist that integration of treatment and prevention become a reality and not a slogan; that "the next wave" of the global epidemic can only be stopped by effective implementation of rights-based programming; and that the next generation of AIDS can only be avoided by measures that will make the rights and lives of women and children central to all our efforts.

The strength of the U.S.-based treatment access movement lies in being part of the global movement, and we must always be self-conscious about how our actions coordinate with the demands and campaigns of activists in the countries most heavily impacted by AIDS. This is increasingly important as the most crucial obstacles to expanded access are now in those countries. Many of the countries which have received Global Fund monies have either not spent it at all or are dramatically behind schedule. Whether this is due to serious problems with implementation, a lack of political commitment or corruption, or other factors, only the people of those countries will be able to hold their governments accountable. Implementation is now the challenge that must be met, and activists in poor and developing countries are critical to moving the roll-out ahead and ensuring that it is done equitably and with input from people with HIV.

The Treatment Action Campaign of South Africa, which has consistently played a leading role in the global movement, recognized this in 2003 and developed a campaign to involve the community in improving the public health services in South Africa. Zackie Achmat, in a speech in New York at that time, gave U.S. activists some salient and strategic advice: "Get your government to send us public health experts but leave the missionaries at home." PEPFAR has resulted in a significant stream of public health experts and an absolute deluge of missionaries. It is our job in the United States to correct the balance.

The global treatment access movement in the United States is based on the experience and lessons of the first generation of AIDS activism that emerged from the gay and lesbian community: remember that every life matters; keep people alive today so that they can benefit from tomorrow's advances; respond with solidarity to efforts to divide us into "innocent victims" and "guilty sinners"; recognize the central role and leadership of people with HIV. Those principles will continue to serve us well as we move forward into the third decade of fighting back against AIDS.

How You Can Become Involved in the Fight against Global AIDS

T he global treatment access movement, and the AIDS activist movement from which it came, have been fueled by the collective action of thousands of people who donated their time, talent, and money to the work. Because of the Internet, it is now possible to think and act *both* locally and globally. Most communities have opportunities to work with local groups of people with HIV and/or other vulnerable populations, and it is possible to be a global treatment or AIDS activist wherever there is a phone and Internet access.

GETTING STARTED

Often the hardest—and most important—part of contributing to an ongoing effort is taking the first step. Every person who has participated in the AIDS and treatment activist movements had to decide how to begin. Here are some suggestions to start the process.

- *Find out more.* Listed below are a few of the thousands of organizations that are active in the struggle. Check out their Web sites, as well as the list of information resources below, and share the news with others.
- *Make a financial contribution.* Most of the organizations listed below rely on the support of voluntary contributions, and won't take money from government or other sources that might compromise their message or actions. Show your support by helping to underwrite their work.
- *Join a listserv.* An excellent way to find out about current problems and campaigns is to join a list of people interested and working on similar issues. Many of the organizations listed below maintain open listservs and advertise how to join them on their Web sites.

- *Join an action.* Among the most important, and overlooked, resources that we all have are our voices and our bodies. Anyone can make a phone call, anyone can wear a message, and anyone can stand in front of a key decision maker and advocate a position. We can all take action, even as we continue to learn more about the issues.
- *Organize with others.* Many of the groups below can help support the organization of a new group, or a new chapter of an existing group. Bring a few friends or people with similar interests together, and discuss whether you want to become an organization.

ACTIVIST AND ADVOCACY ORGANIZATIONS

All of the following organizations are active in the struggle for global and/or U.S. domestic treatment access. This is necessarily an incomplete list, and many of the organizations listed below will also have links to other groups on their Web sites. Consider contacting any of the organizations below as a volunteer or to make a financial contribution.

ACT UP

ACT UP defines itself as a diverse, nonpartisan group of individuals united in anger and committed to direct action to end the AIDS crisis. The best way to learn more about any local ACT UP chapter is to attend a meeting. ACT UP can also provide support to people interested in starting (or reestablishing) a local chapter.

ACT UP EAST BAY

PO Box 8074
Oakland, CA 94662
Email: johnnyi@surfree.com
Phone: 510-841-4339

ACT UP NEW YORK

332 Bleecker Street Suite G5
New York, NY 10014
Web site: www.actupny.org
Phone: 212-966-4873

ACT UP PARIS

BP 287
75525 PARIS Cedex 11
Web site: www.actupparis.org
Phone: 33-1-48-0613-89
Fax: 33-1-48-06-16-74

ACT UP PHILADELPHIA

PO Box 22439 Land Title Station
Philadelphia, PA 19110-2439
Web site: www.critpath.org/actup/
Phone: 215-731-1844
Fax: 215-731-1845

AGUA BUENA HUMAN RIGHTS ASSOCIATION (AGUA BUENA)

Agua Buena is an organization created in response to the AIDS epidemic in
Central America. It has evolved to advocate for access to medical treatment
for PLWHAs in Latin America and the Caribbean.
PO Box 366-2200 Coronado
San Jose, Costa Rica
Phone: 506-234-24-11
Web site: www.aguabuena.org

AMERICAN MEDICAL STUDENTS ASSOCIATION (AMSA)

AMSA sponsors the health professional students' AIDS advocacy network,
which has representatives at medical, public health, and nursing schools
around the United States. They sponsor a number of advocacy events
including (in cooperation with Physicians for Human Rights) a Global
AIDS Advocacy week.
1902 Association Drive
Reston, VA 20191
Web site: www.amsa.org/global/hpsaan.cfm

CENTER FOR HEALTH AND GENDER EQUITY (CHANGE)

CHANGE is a U.S.-based organization that focuses on the effects of U.S.
international policy on the sexual and reproductive rights of women, girls,

and vulnerable populations in Asia, Africa, and Latin America. CHANGE has been an active member in the treatment activist movement, and a leading voice in connecting the ways in which treatment and prevention policies relate to one another.
6930 Carroll Avenue, Suite 910
Takoma Park, MD 20912
Web site: www.genderhealth.org
Phone: 301-270-1182
Fax: 301-270-2052

COMMUNITY HIV/AIDS MOBILIZATION PROJECT (CHAMP)

Led by a founding member of Health GAP and ACT UP Philadelphia, CHAMP is leading a national initiative to build a powerful, community-based movement bridging HIV/AIDS, human rights, and struggles for social and economic justice.
80A 4th Avenue
Brooklyn, NY 11217
Web site: www.aidsinfonyc.org/champ
Phone: 212-437-0254

GLOBAL AIDS ALLIANCE

GAA is a Washington DC–based organization dedicated to a collaborative, aggressive campaign to stop global AIDS. GAA has worked directly on global treatment access and resource mobilization to support it, as well as on debt cancellation and policy change to aid AIDS orphans and vulnerable children.
1225 Connecticut Avenue NW, 4th floor
Washington, DC 20036
Web site: www.globalaidsalliance.org
Phone: 202-296-0260
Fax: 202-296-0261

HEALTH GLOBAL ACCESS PROJECT (HEALTH GAP)

Health GAP is a U.S.-based organization dedicated to eliminating the barriers to global access to affordable medications for people living with HIV/AIDS. The group challenges barriers erected by governments and industry. It also works to ensure that adequate resources are made available to provide for treatment and care and monitors the programs that these resources support.

In New York:
973 St. John's Place #2
Brooklyn NY 11213
Phone: 347-715-5731
In Philadelphia:
4951 Catherine Street
Philadelphia, PA 19143
Phone: 267-475-2645
In San Francisco:
584 Castro Street, #416
San Francisco, CA 94114
Phone: 415-863-4676
Fax: 415-863-4740
Web site: www.healthgap.org

MÉDECINS SANS FRONTIÈRES (DOCTORS WITHOUT BORDERS)

MSF is an international humanitarian agency that provides medical care to
endangered people around the world. Its Campaign for Access to Essential
Medicines works to ensure that the essential drugs for AIDS and other
diseases are made available to the people who need them.
6 East 39th Street, 8th Floor
New York, NY 10016
Web site: www.doctorswithoutborders.org
Phone: 212-655-3764
Fax: 212-6797016

PARTNERS IN HEALTH

Partners in Health is a nonprofit organization that works in Latin America,
the Caribbean, Eastern Europe, and the United States. It seeks to overcome
health problems that conventional wisdom deems "insoluble," and is well-
known within the treatment access movement for its pioneering project in
Haiti that demonstrated that antiretroviral treatment could be successful in
highly impoverished locations.
641 Huntington Avenue
Boston, MA 02115
Web site: www.pih.org
Phone: 617-432-5256

PHYSICIANS FOR HUMAN RIGHTS

Together with Partners in Health, PHR coordinates the Health Action
AIDS Campaign that mobilizes health professionals to support a compre-
hensive AIDS strategy and advocate for funds to fight the disease.
Two Arrow Street, Suite 301
Cambridge, MA 02138
Web site: www.phrusa.org/campaigns/aids/
Phone: 617-301-4200
Fax: 617-301-4250

STUDENT GLOBAL AIDS CAMPAIGN—GLOBAL JUSTICE

The Student Global AIDS Campaign is a U.S.-based network of student
and youth organizations committed to the global fight against AIDS. It
advocates for sufficient resources, effective prevention, and guaranteed
access to AIDS treatment and care.
1225 Connecticut Avenue, Suite 401
Washington, DC 20036
Web site: www.fightglobalaids.org
Phone: 202-296-6727
Fax: 202-296-6728

TREATMENT ACTION CAMPAIGN

The Treatment Action Campaign is a South Africa–based organization
launched in 1998. Its main objective is to promote greater access to AIDS
treatment for all South Africans by raising awareness and understanding
about the availability, affordability, and use of HIV treatments.
TAC National Office
34 Main Road
Mulzenberg 7945
South Africa
Web site: www.tac.org.za
Phone: +27 (21) 788-3507
Fax: +27 (21) 788-3726

WOMEN'S EQUITY IN ACCESS TO CARE AND TREATMENT (WE-ACTX)

WE-ACTx is a U.S.-based organization mobilized to fight the female AIDS pandemic. It is focused primarily on women and girls in East Africa and has begun as its first project a treatment program for women in Rwanda to help genocide rape survivors survive AIDS.
3345 22nd Street
San Francisco, CA 94110
Web site: www.we-actx.org
Phone: 415-648-1728

FOR MORE INFORMATION

The Web sites and materials of the organizations listed above are excellent starting points for gathering more information and educational resources. Below are listed a few more resources that may be helpful.

AIDS EDUCATION GLOBAL INFORMATION SYSTEMS (AEGIS)

Web site: www.aegis.org
This continuously updated clearinghouse of information provides an enormous array of news stories, documents, legal and treatment resources, and an extensive list of links to other resources.

AIDSPAN

Web site: www.aidspan.org
AIDSPAN is a Web site that independently monitors and supports the Global Fund to Fight AIDS, Tuberculosis, and Malaria. It is an excellent source of information on the Global Fund including information about grant rewards. Also publishes the *Global Fund Observer*.

AIDS TREATMENT NEWS

Web site: www.aids.org/atn/
Published twice monthly since 1986, the Web site has a complete archive of every edition. This is an internationally known resource for PLWHAs, providing the latest about treatment—as well as other AIDS news and controversies—in easy to understand and helpful terms.

CENTERS FOR DISEASE CONTROL AND PREVENTION (CDC)

Web site: www.cdc.gov
The CDC is responsible for tracking the HIV/AIDS epidemic in the United States, as well as for prevention activities. Increasingly, it also works with governments in developing countries on these tasks. The Web site is an excellent source of data and statistics regarding HIV infection and AIDS rates in the United States.

COMING TO SAY GOODBYE

Produced by:
Old Dog Documentaries, Inc.
5 W. 19th Street, 3rd Floor
New York, NY 10011-4216
Web site: www.olddogdocumetaries.com
Phone: 212-929-9557
This thirty-minute documentary is a collection of stories about the courageous people living with HIV in Kenya and Tanzania. It also portrays the equally heroic acts of church workers, medical professionals, social workers, and educators working in solidarity with them.

IT'S MY LIFE

Distributed by:
First Run/Icarus Films
32 Court Street, 21st Floor
Brooklyn, NY 11201
Web site: www.frif.com
Phone: 718-488-8900
This is a seventy-two-minute film profiling South Africa's Zackie Achmat, chair of the Treatment Action Campaign (TAC). The film was shot over five months while Zackie was publicly refusing to take antiretroviral drugs until the South African government made them available in the public sector.

PILLS, PROFITS, PROTEST

Distributed by:
Outcast Films
P.O. Box 260
New York, NY 10032
Web site: www.outcast-films.com
Phone: 917-521-2498

This sixty-minute documentary follows the global treatment access movement from the slums of Brazil to villages in Uganda, to the halls of the UN. It includes personal narratives, interviews with key decision makers and activists, and footage of protests and actions to outline the narrative of how the battle for universal treatment has been, and continues to be, waged.

JOINT UNITED NATIONS PROGRAM ON HIV/AIDS (UNAIDS)

Web site: www.unaids.org

UNAIDS is an organization combining contributions from eight United Nations organizations, including the World Health Organization, the World Bank, UNICEF, and others. Its mandate is to promote global action on the AIDS pandemic. The Web site includes many fact sheets and information resources. Every year on December 1 (World AIDS Day) UNAIDS releases an updated report on the global AIDS pandemic.

Notes

Preface

1. Doug McAdam (1982) *Political Process and the Development of Black Insurgency, 1930–1970*, Chicago, Illinois: University of Chicago Press.
2. Margaret Keck and Kathryn Sikkink (1998) *Activists beyond Borders: Advocacy Networks in International Politics*, Ithaca, New York: Cornell University Press.

Part I. Introduction

1. Doug McAdam (1982) *Political Process and the Development of Black Insurgency, 1930–1970*, Chicago, Illinois: University of Chicago Press. For further discussion of the political process model, see also: Jeff Goodwin and James M. Jasper (Eds.) (2004) *Rethinking Social Movements: Structure, Meaning, and Emotion*, Lanham, Maryland: Rowman & Littlefield Publishers.

Chapter 1. ACTION=LIFE: Responding to AIDS on the Home Front

1. For more on the antibiotics revolution, see Eric Lax (2004) *The Mold in Dr. Florey's Coat: The Story of the Penicillin Miracle*, New York: Henry Holt.
2. World Health Organization (undated) "Smallpox"; accessed at www.who.int/mediacentre/factsheets/smallpox/en/ on June 1, 2005.
3. Centers for Disease Control and Prevention (1981) "*Pneumocystis* Pneumonia—Los Angeles," *Morbidity and Mortality Report*, 30: 250–252, June 5.
4. Centers for Disease Control and Prevention (1981) "Kaposi's Sarcoma and *Pneumocystis* Pneumonia among Homosexual Men—New York and California," *Morbidity and Mortality Report*, 30: 305–307, July 3.

5. Cited in Randy Shilts (1987) *And the Band Played On: Politics, People and the AIDS Epidemic*, New York: St. Martin's Press.

6. Cited in Mark Thompson (Ed.) (1994) *Long Road to Freedom: The* Advocate *History of the Gay and Lesbian Movement*, New York: St. Martin's Press, p. 195.

7. Raymond A. Smith (2001) "Print Journalism," in R. Smith (Ed.) *The Encylcopedia of AIDS*, New York: Penguin, pp. 307–310.

8. Cited in Shilts, op. cit., pp. 450–451.

9. *Longtime Companion*, directed by Norman Rene, was released by the Samuel Goldwyn Company and American Playhouse in 1990.

10. Richard Colvin (2001) "People with Hemophilia," in R. Smith (Ed.) *The Encyclopedia of AIDS*, New York: Penguin, pp. 307–310.

11. Susan Chambre (1991) "The Volunteer Response to the AIDS Epidemic in New York City: Implications for Research on Voluntarism," *Nonprofit and Voluntary Sector Quarterly*, 20(3): 279–280.

12. Philip M. Kayal (1993) *Bearing Witness: Gay Men's Health Crisis and the Politics of AIDS*, Boulder, Colorado: Westview Press, p. 14.

13. Ibid., p. 15.

14. Michael Callan and Dan Turner (1997) "A History of the People with AIDS Self-Empowerment Movement," *Body Positive Magazine*, 10(12): 12–25, December.

15. Ibid.

16. Ibid.

17. Ibid.

18. Ibid.

19. Susan Chambre (1996) "Uncertainty, Diversity, and Change: The AIDS Community in New York City," *Research in Community Sociology*, 6: 161.

20. Maxine Wolfe (1997) "This Is about People Dying: The Tactics of Early ACT UP and Lesbian Avengers in New York City," based on interviews with Laraine Sommella, in Gordon Brent Ingram, Anne-Marie Bouthillette, and Yolanda Retter (Eds.) *Queers in Space: Communities, Public Places, Sites of Resistance*, Seattle, Washington: Bay Press.

21. Larry Kramer (1983) "1,112 and Counting," *The New York Native*, March 1983, reprinted in Chris Bull (Ed.) (2003) *While the World Sleeps: Writing from the First Twenty Years of the Global AIDS Plague*, New York: Thunder's Mouth Press, pp. 18–19.

22. Wolfe, op. cit.

23. Ibid.

24. Ronald Medley (2001) "Demonstrations and Direct Actions," in R. Smith (Ed.) *The Encyclopedia of AIDS*, New York: Penguin, pp. 199–203.

25. *Bowers v. Hardwick* (1986) 478 US 186.

26. Deborah Gould (2001) "Rock the Boat, Don't Rock the Boat Baby: Ambivalence and the Emergence of Militant AIDS Activism," in Jeff Goodwin, James M. Jasper, and Francesca Polletta (Eds.) *Passionate Politics: Emotions and Social Movements*, Chicago: University of Chicago Press, p. 166.

27. Maer Roshan (2002) "ACT UP," *The Advocate*, November 12; accessed at www.advocate.com/html/stories/876/876_actup.asp on December 14, 2004.

28. ACT UP New York (1987) "Flyer of the First ACT UP Action, March 24, 1987, Wall Street, New York City"; accessed at www.actupny.org/documents/1stFlyer.html on October 25, 2004.

29. Medley, op. cit.

30. Wolfe, op. cit.

31. Deborah B. Gould (undated) "Life during Wartime: Emotions and the Development of ACT UP"; accessed at http://www.actupny.org/indexfolder/gould_s02.pdf#search='life%20during%20wartime%20aids%20gould' on October 25, 2004.

32. Cited in Deborah R. Gould (2004) "Passionate Political Processes: Bringing Emotions Back into the Study of Social Movements," in Jeff Goodwin and James M. Jasper (Eds.) *Rethinking Social Movements: Structure, Meaning, and Emotion*, Lanham, Maryland: Rowman & Littlefield Publishers, p. 8.

33. ACT UP New York (undated) "ACT UP Capsule History 1992"; accessed at www.actupny.org/documents/cron-92.html on October 25, 2004.

34. ACT UP New York (undated) "How to Start an ACT UP Chapter"; accessed at www.actupny.org/documents/start_chapter.html on October 25, 2004.

35. ACT UP New York (undated) "New Members Packet"; accessed at www.actupny.org/documents/newmem.html on October 25, 2004.

36. ACT UP New York (1987) "Original Working Document"; accessed at www.actupny.org/documents/firstworkingdoc.html on October 25, 2004.

37. ACT UP New York (undated) "Monday Night Meetings"; accessed at www.actupny.org/documents/newmem1.html on October 25, 2004.

38. Cited in Gould, op. cit. (note 32), p. 8.

39. Gilbert Elbaz (1992) "The Sociology of AIDS Activism: The Case of ACT UP/New York, 1987–1992," unpublished dissertation, City University of New York, p. 65.

40. ACT UP New York (undated) "Actions and Zaps"; accessed at www.actupny.org/documents/newmem2.html on October 25, 2004.

41. Ibid.

42. Ibid.

43. Aldyn McKean (undated) "Why We Get Arrested"; accessed at www.actupny.org/documents/whywe%20get.html on October 25, 2004.

44. Ibid.

45. Wolfe, op. cit.

46. Clara Orban (2001) "Visual Arts," in R. Smith (Ed.) *The Encyclopedia of AIDS*, New York: Penguin, pp. 738–741.

47. Steven Epstein (1996) *Impure Science: AIDS, Activism, and the Politics of Knowledge*, Berkeley, California: University of California Press, p. 9.

48. Ibid., p. 336.

49. Vito Russo (1988) "Why We Fight," video transcript of speech delivered at the ACT UP demonstration in Albany, New York, May 9, 1988, and the ACT UP demonstration at the Department of Health and Human Services, Washington DC, October 10, 1988; accessed at www.actupny.org/documents/whfight.html on October 25, 2004.

50. Jon Greenberg (1992) "ACT UP Explained"; accessed at www.actupny.org/documents/greenbergau.html on October 25, 2004.

51. ACT UP New York, op. cit. (note 33)

52. ACT UP Boston (1990) "Up Till Now Survival Has Prevented Us from Living," *Attitude!*, January, p. 1.

53. ACT UP New York, op. cit. (note 33)

54. Ibid.

55. ACT UP Milwaukee (undated) "ACT UP/Milwaukee, Records 1990–96, Administrative History," University of Wisconsin, Madison, Manuscript Collection 203; accessed at www.uwm.edu/edu/libraries/arch/findaids/uwmmss203.htm on December 14, 2004.

56. ACT UP New York, op. cit. (note 33)

57. Ibid.

58. Ibid.

59. Ibid.

60. Ibid.

61. Ibid.

62. Ibid.

63. Epstein, op. cit., pp. 338–350.

64. Lawrence K. Altman (1993) "Government Panel on HIV Finds the Prospect for Treatment Bleak," *The New York Times*, June 29, p. C3.

65. The New York Times Editorial Board (1993) "The Unyielding AIDS Epidemic," *The New York Times*, June 17, p. A4.

66. Altman, op. cit.

67. Susan Stryker (undated) "Queer Nation," online entry in *glbtq: An Encyclopedia of Gay, Lesbian, Bisexual, Transgender and Queer Culture*; accessed at www.glbtq.com/social-sciences/queer_nation.html on December 14, 2004.

68. Raymond A. Smith and Donald P. Haider-Markel (2002) *Gay and Lesbian Americans and Political Participation*, Santa Barbara, California: ABC-CLIO, pp. 46–50.

69. Craig Rimmerman (2001) "ACT UP," in R. Smith (Ed.) *The Encylcopedia of AIDS*, New York: Penguin, pp. 3–7.

70. Survive AIDS (2000) "A Letter to the Community," March 21; accessed at http://www.actupny.org/indexfolder/actupgg.html on July 15, 2004.

71. Larry Kramer (1990) "A Manhattan Project for AIDS," *The New York Times*, July 16, reprinted in Chris Bull (Ed.) (2003) *While the World Sleeps: Writing from the First Twenty Years of the Global AIDS Plague*, New York: Thunder's Mouth Press, p. 61.

72. ACT UP New York, op. cit. (note 33)
73. Ibid.
74. Jeffry Schmalz (1993) "Whatever Happened to AIDS?," *The New York Times Magazine*, November 28, reprinted in Chris Bull (Ed.) (2003) *While the World Sleeps: Writing from the First Twenty Years of the Global AIDS Plague*, New York: Thunder's Mouth Press, p. 246.

Chapter 2. Bridging the Gap: Mobilizing Global Response

1. George Manos, Leonardo Negron, and Tim Horn (2001) "Antiviral Drugs," in R. Smith (Ed.) *The Encyclopedia of AIDS*, New York: Penguin, pp. 51–53.
2. Ibid.
3. Wei, X. et al. (1995) "Viral Dynamics in Human Immunodeficiency Virus Type-1 Infection," *Nature*, 375(6510): 123–126.
4. Tim Horn (2001) "Drug Resistance," in R. Smith (Ed.) *The Encyclopedia of AIDS*, New York: Penguin, pp. 218–219.
5. Manos et al., op. cit.
6. Centers for Disease Control and Prevention (1999) *HIV/AIDS Surveillance Report*, 11(1): 32–37.
7. Elizabeth Heubeck (2003) "ADAP in Peril," *Numedx*, 5(1): 29, Spring/ Summer 2003.
8. Centers for Disease Control and Prevention (1992) "1993 Revised Classification System for HIV Infection and Expanded Surveillance Definition for AIDS among Adolescents and Adults," *Morbidity and Mortality Weekly Report*, 41: 1–19, December 3.
9. UNAIDS (2000) "Report of the State of the Epidemic"; accessed at www. unaids.org on July 4, 2005.
10. Ibid.
11. Ibid.
12. World Bank Group—Data and Statistics; accessed at http:// www.worldbank.org/data/countryclass/classgroups.htm on July 4, 2005.
13. Eileen Stillwagon (2002) "HIV/AIDS in Africa: Fertile Terrain," *Journal of Development Studies*, 38(2): 5.
14. James G. Kublin et al. (2005) "Effect of *Plasmodium falciparum* on Concentration on Hiv-1 RNA in the Blood of Adults in Rural Malawi: A Prospective Cohort Study," *The Lancet*, 365(9455): 233–240, January 15; accessed at www.thelancet.com on July 4, 2005.
15. UNAIDS (2001) "Gender and HIV: The Facts about Women and HIV/ AIDS," p. 1; accessed at http://www.unaids.org/html/pub/Publications/ Fact-sheets02/FS_Gender_en_pdf.htm on February 18, 2004.
16. Human Rights Watch (2003) "Policy Paralysis: A Call for Action on HIV/ Aids-Related Human Rights Abuses against Women and Girls in Africa," p. 17; accessed at http://www.hrw.org/reports/2003/africa1203.pdf. on February 18, 2004.

17. Noleen Heyzer (2001) Address to the United Nations General Assembly Special Session on HIV/AIDS, New York, p. 2; accessed at http://www.un.org/ga/aids/statements/docs/unifemE.html on September 25, 2002.

18. Tony Barnett and Alan Whiteside (2003) *AIDS in the Twenty-first Century: Disease and Globalization*, London: Palgrave Macmillan, p. 190.

19. Tina Rosenberg (2001) "How to Solve the World's AIDS Crisis," *New York Times Magazine*, January 28.

20. Jan Aart Scholte (2000) *Globalization: A Critical Introduction*, New York: St. Martin's Press, p. 44–46.

21. Donna Rae, Palmer, Paul Davis, David Hoos, John James, and Toby Casper (1999) "Globalization and Unequal Access to Health Care: Resources for People with AIDS and Other Life-Threatening Illnesses," Health GAP, November 29, p. 6.

22. World Health Organization (1995) "Trade-Related Aspects of Intellectual Property Rights (TRIPS)"; accessed at www.wto.org/english/docs_e/legal_e/27-trips_o1_e.htm on June 5, 2005.

23. Susan K. Sell (2003) *Private Power, Public Law: The Globalization of Intellectual Property Rights*, Cambridge: Cambridge University Press, pp. 1–2.

24. Ibid., pp. 7–8.

25. World Health Organization, op. cit.

26. Palmer et al., op. cit., p. 6.

27. Ibid.

28. Arnold S. Relman and Marcia Angell (2002) "America's Other Drug Problem," *The New Republic*, no. 4587, December 16, p. 28.

29. Jonathan Mann (1996) "The Future of the AIDS Movement"; accessed at www.aids.harvard.edu/publications/har/spring_1999/Spring99-7.html on May 6, 2002.

30. Peter Piot (1998) "Bridging the Gap"; accessed at www.unaids.org/whatsnew/speeches/end/12thconf.html on April 27, 2002.

31. Gillian Murphy (2002) "In Search of Solidarity," *Body Positive Magazine*, 15(6): 23–28.

32. Interview with Alan Berkman by Raymond Smith on February 21, 2002.

33. Ibid.

34. Ibid.

35. Ibid.

36. Rosenberg, op. cit., pp. 26 ff.

37. John James (1998) personal e-mail sent on September 8, 1998 to James Love; provided by John James.

38. John James (1998) "GATT and the Gap: How to Save Lives," *AIDS Treatment News*, November 20.

39. James Love (undated) Homepage: "About James Love"; accessed at www.cptech.org/jamie/ on September 20, 2003.

40. John James (1999) "Compulsory Licensing: Bridging the Gap—Treatment Access in Developing Countries: Interview with James Love," *AIDS Treatment News*, March 5.

41. Alan Berkman (1998) "From Geneva to Durban: Solidarity Bridges the Gap," unpublished manuscript, October.

42. Ibid., pp. 2–3.

43. Interview with Alan Berkman, op. cit.

44. Ibid.

45. Health GAP (2002) "About Health GAP"; accessed at www.healthgap.org/hgap/about.html on July 17, 2002.

46. Ibid.

47. Ibid.

48. Frank Bruni (1997) "ACT UP Doesn't Much, Anymore: A Decade-Old Activism of Unmitigated Gall Is Fading" *New York Times,* March 21; accessed at www.glaxowellcome.ch/gw/dt/news/mar97/21397.141033.html on March 2, 2002.

49. Associated Press (2001) "AIDS Advocacy Group Expands Interest," May 12; accessed at http://projects.is.asu.edu/pipermail/hpn/2001-may/00383.html on March 2, 2002.

50. PhillyMag.com (2001) "Send Bohos, Nuts, and Addicts"; accessed at www.phillymag.om/archives/2001nov/actup_1.html on October 25, 2004.

51. Ibid.

52. Associated Press, op. cit.

53. Eric Sawyer (2002) "An ACT UP Founder 'Acts Up' for Africa's Access to Treatment," introductory notes, in B. Shephard and R. Hayduk (Eds.) *From ACT UP to the WTO: Urban Protest and Community Building in the Era of Globalization,* New York: Verso, p. 88.

54. Interview with Sharonann Lynch by Raymond Smith on February 16, 2003.

55. Health GAP (undated) "Health GAP Timeline: Direct Actions, Advocacy, and Response," unpublished document, January 1999–December 2000.

56. Health GAP (2000) "ACT UP Disrupts House Vote"; accessed at www.agrnews.org/issues/69/nationalnews.html on March 2, 2002.

57. ACT UP (1999) "Gore Concedes to Life-Saving Compromise on SA Drug Policy," ACT UP press release, September 17, 2002; accessed at www.globaltreatmentaccess.org/content/press_releases/99/091977_AU on March, 2, 2002.

58. HIV/AIDS Treatment Action Campaign (TAC) (1999) "Open Letter Concerning United States Pressure on the South African Government on Compulsory Licensing and Parallel Imports," July 5.

59. Mark Weisbrot (1999) "Shaming the Powerful" Knight Ridder/Tribune Media Services, September 22, 1999; accessed at www.cepr.net/columns/weisbrot/shaming_the_powerful.htm on March 2, 2002.

60. Robert Weissman (1999) "AIDS Drugs for Africa: Grassroots Pressure Overcomes US-Industry 'Full Court Press' to Block South Africa's

Affordable Medicine Program," *Multinational Monitor*, 20(9); accessed at www.essential.org/monitor/mm1999/99sept/aids.htm on March 2, 2002.

61. Interview with Alan Berkman, op. cit.
62. Interview with Mark Milano by Raymond Smith on February 24, 2004.
63. Ibid.
64. ACT UP New York and ACT UP Philadelphia (1999) "AIDS Activists Hit Al Gore Three Times in Two Days: Vice President Dumbfounded, Confused, Unable to Respond," ACT UP press release, June 18.
65. Interview with Alan Berkman, op. cit.
66. ACT UP Philadelphia (1999) "Al Gore's 'Apartheid 2000' Campaign Comes to Philadelphia," ACT UP press release, June 23.
67. Sonya Ross (1999) "Gore Caught in AIDS Activist Rift," Associated Press, June 30; accessed at www.glinn.com/news/aidsact.htm on March 2, 2002.
68. Ibid.
69. Greg Behrman (2004) *The Invisible People: How the U.S. Has Slept Through the Global AIDS Pandemic, the Greatest Humanitarian Catastrophe of Our Time*, New York: Free Press, p. 158.
70. ACT UP Philadelphia and ACT UP New York (1999) "U.S. Trade Representative Barshefsky Gets Bon Voyage to WTO," ACT UP press release, November 17.
71. Behrman, op. cit., p. 157.
72. Ibid., p. 158.
73. Al Gore (2000) "Remarks as Prepared for Delivery by Vice President Al Gore, UN Security Council Session on AIDS in Africa, January 10, 2002," the White House, Office of the Vice President; accessed at www.un.int/usa/00_002.htm on March 2, 2002.
74. Ibid.
75. Behrman, op. cit., p. 150.
76. CNN (2000) "US to Seek $100 Million in Global Anti-AIDS Effort," CNN.com, January 10; accessed at www.cnn.com/2000/us/01/10/aids.africa.01 on March 2, 2002.
77. Kevin Danaher and Roger Burbach (Eds.) (2000) *Globalize This! The Battle against the World Trade Organization and Corporate Rule*, Monroe, Maine: Common Courage Press, p. 7.
78. Paul Hawken (2000) "Skeleton Woman Visits Seattle," in Kevin Danaher and Roger Burbach (Eds.) *Globalize This! The Battle against the World Trade Organization and Corporate Rule*, Monroe, Maine: Common Courage Press, p. 15.
79. Benjamin Shephard and Ronald Hayduk (Eds.) (2002) *From ACT UP to the WTO: Urban Protest and Community Building in the Era of Globalization*, New York: Verso.
80. Benjamin Shephard (2002) "Introductory Notes on the Trail from ACT UP to the WTO," in Benjamin Shephard and Ronald Hayduk (Eds.) *From ACT*

UP to the WTO: Urban Protest and Community Building in the Era of Globalization, New York: Verso, p. 13.

Part II. Introduction

1. Margaret E. Keck and Kathryn Sikkink (1998) *Activists beyond Borders: Advocacy Networks in International Politics*, Ithaca, New York: Cornell University Press, pp. 8, 9.
2. Doug McAdam (1982) *Political Process and the Development of Black Insurgency, 1930–1970*, Chicago, Illinois: University of Chicago Press, p. 42.
3. Ibid., p. 43.
4. Keck and Sikkink, op. cit., p. 1.
5. Ibid., p. 9.
6. Ibid., p. 12.
7. Ibid., pp. 40–41.
8. Clifford Bob (2002) "Merchants of Morality," *Foreign Policy*, March: 36–46.

Chapter 3. Many Places, One Goal: Connecting Global Actors

1. Edwin Cameron (2000) "The Deafening Silence of AIDS," Jonathan Mann Memorial Lecture, Thirteenth International AIDS Conference, Durban, South Africa, July 10.
2. AIDS Consortium Homepage; accessed at http://www.aidsconsortium.org.za on July 16, 2005.
3. Claire Keeton (2001) "S. African's Treatment Action Campaign Advances Fight against AIDS," *Agence France Presse*, March 21.
4. Information about these actions was taken from Human Rights Watch (2004) *Deadly Delay: South Africa's Efforts to Prevent HIV in Survivors of Sexual Violence*, 16(3A): 18–20, March, and Patricia Siplon (2002) *AIDS and the Policy Struggle in the United States*, Washington DC: Georgetown University Press, p. 111.
5. Rosalind Petchesky (2003) *Global Prescriptions: Gendering Health and Human Rights*, London and New York: Zed Books, p. 88.
6. Richard Parker (2003) "Building the Foundations for the Response to HIV/AIDS in Brazil: The Development of HIV/AIDS Policy, 1982–1996" *Divulgaceo em Saude para Debate*, 27: 143–183.
7. Ibid.
8. Ibid., pp. 158–159.
9. Petchesky, op. cit., p. 99.
10. Parker, op. cit., p. 160.
11. Raymond A. Smith (2004) "Organizing for Access: The Agua Buena Human Rights Association, *Body Positive*," 17(1): 30–31.

12. Human Rights Watch (2004) *Not Enough Graves: The War on Drugs, HIV/AIDS and the Violation of Human Rights*, July.

13. Karen Kaplan (2002) "The Body: Interview with Paisan Tan-ud," *GMHC Treatment Issues*, 16(11), November; accessed at http://www.thebody.com/gmhc/issues/nov02/tan-ud.html on February 14, 2004.

14. Khalil Elouardighi, e-mail interview with Raymond Smith and Patricia Siplon on February 24, 2005.

15. Interview with Pauline Ngunjiri by Patricia Siplon at the United Nations General Assembly Special Session on HIV/AIDS, New York City, June 26, 2001.

16. Andrew Maykuth (2001) "Drug Industry Says South Africa Repeatedly Spurned Offers to Discount AIDS Medicine," *Philadelphia Inquirer*, April 18, p. A02.

17. Rachel L. Swarns (2001) "Drug Makers Drop South Africa Suit over AIDS Medicine," *New York Times*, April 20, p. A1.

18. Samuel Siringi (2001) "Generic Drugs Battle Moves from South Africa to Kenya," *The Lancet*, 357(9268): 1600.

19. The Nation (2001) "HIV/AIDS Drug Imports Blocked by WTO," *Africa News*, October 10.

20. See, for example, Geoff Dyer, David Pilling, Vanessa Valkin, and Frances Williams (2001) "US Climbs Down over Brazil's Patent Law," *Financial Times* (London), June 26, p. 8; and Peter Capella (2001) "Brazil Wins HIV Concession from US: Complaint to WTO on Patent Law Withdrawn," *The Guardian*, June 26, p. 18.

21. Richard Kim (2001) "Stop Global AIDS," *The Nation*, June 23; accessed at www.thenation.com on August 23, 2001.

22. Theresa Agovino (2001) "Delegate: AIDS Goal Too Ambitious," Associated Press, June 25.

23. Derek Hodel (2004) "At the Crossroads: A Study of Federal HIV/AIDS Advocacy," New York: Ford Foundation; accessed at http://www.fcaaids.org/publications/HIV_entire_book.pdf on January 6, 2005.

24. Ibid., p. 39.

Chapter 4. Win Some, Keep Going: Sustaining Global AIDS Treatment Activism

1. John A. Jernigan et al. (2001) "Bioterrorism-Related Inhalational Anthrax: The First 10 Cases Reported in the United States," *Emerging Infectious Diseases*, 7(6), November–December.

2. Edward Walsh and Carol D. Leonnig (2001) "Anthrax Is Found in House Building: Hill Leaders Ponder a Return to Schedule," *The Washington Post*, October 21, p. A01.

3. Mary Dalrymple (2002) "Senate Observes Anniversary of Anthrax Attack on Daschle Staff," *CQ Monitor News*, October 15.

4. "Ciprofloxin Quotes," a compilation on the Web site of the Consumer Project on Technology; accessed at www.cptech.org on July 15, 2004.

5. Anthony York (2001) "Is It Time to Bust the Cipro Patent?," Salon.com, October 18; accessed on July 15, 2004.

6. Amy Harmon and Robert Pear (2001) "Canada Overrides Patent for Cipro to Treat Anthrax," *The New York Times*, October 19.

7. Information on the Global Fund's operation was taken from the Web site of the Global Fund (www.theglobalfund.org) and of Aidspan, (www.Aidspan. org), an independent monitoring organization.

8. Guy De Jonquieres and Frances Williams (2001) "Global Activists Adopt New Tactics: Switch to Behind-the-Scenes Influence," *Financial Times*, November 12.

9. Andrew Pollack (2001) "Much of the Policy Criticism Aimed at U.S. Turns Muted," *The New York Times*, September 27.

10. Jonquieres and Williams, op. cit.

11. Geoff Winestock and Helene Cooper (2001) "Deal Will Allow Poor Nations to Ignore Patents to Meet Public-Health Needs," *Wall Street Journal*, November 14.

12. The text of the Declaration on the TRIPS agreement and public health (the "Doha Declaration") can be found on the WTO's Web site at http:// www.wto.org/english/thewto_e/minist_e/min01_e/mindecl_trips_e.htm; last accessed on July 15, 2004.

13. Donald G. MacNeil Jr. (2001) "Coca-Cola Joins AIDS Fight in Africa," *New York Times*, June 21, p. 8; Betsy McKay (2001) "Coca-Cola to Tap Its Marketing Muscle to Help Fight AIDS Epidemic in Africa," *Wall Street Journal*, June 20.

14. Agence France Press (2002) "Protests Mark AIDS Conference for Third Day Running," July 10.

15. Interview with T. Richard Corcoran by Patricia Siplon on June 18, 2005, New York City.

16. David Brown (2002) "Loud Protesters Drown Out Thompson Speech at International AIDS Conference," *Washington Post*, July 10, p. A02.

17. Jennifer Smith (2002) "ACT UP Protests Coke's 'medical apartheid,'" *Southern Voice*, July 26, p. 5.

18. Ann Carrns (2002) "Coke to Help African Bottlers Include AIDS Care in Benefits," *Wall Street Journal*, September 27.

19. Greg Behrman (2004) *The Invisible People: How the U.S. Has Slept Through the Global AIDS Pandemic, the Greatest Humanitarian Catastrophe of Our Time*, New York: Free Press, p. 273.

20. Ellen't Hoen (2004) "Statement from MSF at the Conference on Fixed Dose Combination (FDC) Drug Products: Scientific and Technical Issues Related to Safety, Quality and Effectiveness," March 20, Gabarone, Botswana.

21. Abner Mason (2004) "The False Promise of Untested AIDS Drugs," *San Francisco Chronicle*, March 29; Robert Goldberg (2004) "Activists against

Africa," *Washington Times*, April 8; and James K. Glassman (2004) "Bush Critics Imperil Africa's AIDS Victims," *Newsday*, April 13.

22. Daniel Wolfe (2004) "Condemned to Death: Thanks to the Drug War, a Global AIDS Epidemic is Exploding among Injection Drug Users," *The Nation*, April 26.

23. Sarah Bosley (2004) "Anger at US Ban on AIDS Scientists: Bangkok Conference Forced to Cancel Meetings and Retract Papers After Authors Stopped from Attending," *The Guardian*, July 12. See also: Katherine Stapp (2004) "US Retreat from AIDS Meet," *IPS*, July 9.

24. Taken from the Web site http://www/bureaucrash.com/ on April 5, 2005.

25. Allison Dinsmore, e-mail communication on April 5, 2005. The film of the counterprotest and written accounts of the "crashers" may be viewed at the Web site http://www.bureaucrash.com; accessed on April 5, 2005.

26. In fact, an independent study verifies the safety of the composition of the medicines in question. See Geethaa Ramachandran, Elke Perloff, Lisa von Moltke, Soumyaa Swaminathan, Christine Wanke, and David Greenblatt (2004) "Analysis of Generic Antiretroviral Formulations Manufactured in India," *AIDS*, 18(10): 1482–1484, July 2. The authors are grateful to Richard Jefferys for posting this information.

27. Kaiser Family Foundation (2004) "Waiting for AIDS Medications in the United States: An Analysis of ADAP Waiting Lists," HIV/AIDS Policy Fact Sheet, December; accessed at http://www.kff.org on April 8, 2005.

28. The Consumer Project on Technology (CPT) has been an active and vocal participant in the debates over the high prices of patented medication. CPT maintains a Web page on the Norvir issue, from which this information was taken; accessed at http://www.cpt.org/ip/health/aids/norvir.html on March 1, 2004.

29. Lauran Neergaard (2004) "Government Won't Intervene in Price of AIDS Drug," *Associated Press*, August 4.

Conclusion

1. Gardiner Harris (2004) "Price of AIDS Drug Intensifies Debate on Legal Imports," *New York Times*, April 14, p. A1.

2. Gregg Gonsalves (2005) "It Ain't What You Do but the Way You Do It: Ten Points on International AIDS Treatment Activism," speech delivered at "Realising the Right to Health: A Global South Dialogue on HIV/AIDS & Access to Treatment," March 18–21, 2005, Mumbai, India.

3. Raymond W. Copson (2000) "AIDS in Africa," Congressional Research Service, issue brief, October 20, pp. 10–11.

Index

About the Authors

RAYMOND A. SMITH is Adjunct Assistant Professor of Political Science at Columbia University and New York University. He is editor of the award-winning *Encyclopedia of AIDS*, general editor of the book series "Political Participation in America," coauthor of *Gay and Lesbian Americans and Political Participation*, and coauthor of *HIV Treatments and Mental Health*. He has served as editor of the community-based HIV/AIDS magazine *Body Positive*, as a researcher at the HIV Center for Clinical and Behavioral Studies, and as research director of the National Alliance of State and Territorial AIDS Directors.

PATRICIA D. SIPLON is Associate Professor of Political Science at Saint Michael's College in Colchester, Vermont. She is the author of *AIDS and the Policy Struggle in the United States*. She has conducted research and done advocacy work on HIV/AIDS politics and policy in the United States and East Africa, most recently as a Fulbright Africa Regional Research Award recipient in Tanzania in 2005.